LIFE AFTER NINETY

Long life, including particularly, the factors which might promote it, is of perennial interest to human beings, but the circumstances of very old people less so. Whilst there is much discussion about ageing in today's society, there is less willingness to examine the assumptions which underpin our attitudes towards old age. These assumptions are based on a variety of contradictory positive and negative sentiments which coalesce into stereotypes.

The very old represent the fastest growing section of the population of most western societies. Reactions by public and politicians alike are often marked by alarm and dismay. It is assumed that the hallmark of very old age is decrepitude, and that, consequently, demands on services will be unmanageable. The very old are thus portrayed as a burden to themselves and others.

In *Life After Ninety* Michael Bury and Anthea Holme have surveyed and interviewed just under 200 individuals, living at home and in communal establishments, which has enabled them to present a unique picture of the health, quality of life, and social circumstances of the very old. Longevity and the factors which promote it are also discussed, and throughout the book the concept of the 'life course' is employed, which brings together the biographical experiences of individuals, and the changing historical circumstances of the twentieth century, through which they have lived.

Though poor health and unhappiness do mar the lives of some individuals and their carers, the book also shows that a good quality of life is often possible in very old age, and that life after ninety can involve both contentment and dignity.

Although this study is presented with the general reader in mind, *Life After Ninety* will be of interest to all those concerned with the elderly, and will be of particular interest to social policy-makers, social workers, geriatricians, doctors, nurses and other care staff. It will also be of particular value to lecturers and students on courses in social gerontology and medical sociology.

Michael Bury is Senior Lecturer in Sociology, and Anthea Holme is a Research Officer, in the Department of Sociology at Royal Holloway and Bedford New College, University of London. They are both experienced social researchers and have published widely in the fields of health, ageing, and sociology.

LIFE AFTER NINETY

Michael Bury
and
Anthea Holme

Foreword by Margot Jefferys

ROUTLEDGE

London and New York

6003567407

First published in 1991
by Routledge
11 New Fetter Lane, London EC4P 4EE

Simultaneously published in the USA and Canada
by Routledge
a division of Routledge, Chapman and Hall Inc.
29 West 35th Street, New York, NY 10001

© 1991 Michael Bury and Anthea Holme

Typeset by Witwell Ltd, Southport .
Printed and bound in Great Britain by
Biddles Ltd, Guildford and King's Lynn

British Library Cataloguing in Publication Data
Bury, Michael, *1945–*
Life after ninety.
1. Old age
I. Title   II. Holme, Anthea
305.26

Library of Congress Cataloging in Publication Data
Bury, Michael, 1945–
Life after ninety/by Michael Bury and Anthea Holme.
p.   cm.
Includes index.
Includes bibliographical references.
1. Aged–Great Britain–Social conditions.   2. Old age–Great
Britain.   3. Longevity–Great Britain.   4. Life cycle, Human.
I. Holme, Anthea.   II. Title.
HQ1064.G7B85   1990   90–35825
305.26'0941–dc20   CIP

ISBN 0–415–04165–1

CONTENTS

FOREWORD

At the end of the nineteenth century, the threats to social order appeared to contemporaries to come from internecine competition among advancing industrial nations for possession of the 'virgin' territories of the continents in the southern hemisphere, as well as from the demands for a larger share of the product of their labour by the proletariats which industrialization and urbanization had spawned. Earlier Malthusian concerns that uncontrolled population growth would outstrip food production had largely disappeared with the opening up of agricultural production on a grand scale in the Americas and Australasia, and the development of maritime transport capacity including refrigeration. Simultaneously, signs that birth as well as death was controllable and that lower fertility benefited those individuals and societies where it was accomplished voluntarily rather than as a result of malnutrition and premature death sustained optimism about the future.

As the twentieth century nears its end, the contemporary spectres which haunt us are markedly different. We are now afraid that the vast technological achievements of the century, fuelled by economic imperatives as well as scientific advances, will, paradoxically, themselves be the means of destruction, not merely of the social orders which have evolved over centuries but, potentially, of human life itself.

Population pressures on resources have also, once again, re-surfaced as a matter of serious debate. The fear is expressed in responsible circles that rapid population explosions in the less technologically developed parts of the world will not only lead to mass starvation in those countries but have knock-on and possibly equally disastrous effects on the rest of the world, which will not be able to insulate itself from involvement.

A parallel contemporary concern in most industrial nations,

however, is a domestic one. It arises from what has been described as the 'greying' of the population, that is the growing number of individuals from each birth generation who survive, not only to an age when they are able, indeed encouraged, to retire from active involvement in the formal productive economy, but, increasingly, into their eighties, nineties and hundreds. Since they are no longer engaged in productive enterprise, they are economically dependent on those who are. And as they age, there is a strong likelihood that they will become physically dependent on others to maintain the minimal activities required to sustain daily living activities.

Ironically, the twentieth-century conquest of premature death is now portrayed as having created an economic burden on the resources of society of such gross dimensions that it threatens the well-being, not merely of the very old themselves, but of younger generations who have to make sacrifices to serve their voracious needs for health and welfare services. To this economic burden must be added the emotional costs borne by those who, as a result of accepting kinship ties and obligations to their elders, have to sacrifice their own interests, or those of younger kin, the children with whom the future lies. Indeed, some of the media discussion of the issues surrounding an ageing population can give the impression that the old – and especially the very old – threaten to replace lager louts and loony lefts as those likely to lead to a breakdown in the social order.

A whole new series of expressions reflect these concerns, if not panics. They have entered, if not everyday popular vocabulary, at least the political discourse of our time. Demographers and economists talk about the *dependency ratio*, social policy analysts about *generational equity*, political economists about *structured dependency* and sociologists about *the social construction of age* and *ageism*. Ageing as a process and old age as both a state of being and a socially constructed concept have become subjects for research in the fast burgeoning field of academic social gerontology. Empirical research, directed largely to identifying needs of older people for various kinds of health and social support services and to determining how these needs can be met, receives as much, if not more, support from government and voluntary funding bodies than does research related to other potentially dependent and vulnerable groups.

Hitherto, however, it has been noticeable that most of the research undertaken in the UK and the USA, as well as in other countries, has tended to take as its study population, those of pensionable age and over, a section of the population with an age span of well over 30 years.

In the analysis of survey results, a distinction is now commonly made between those over or under the age of 75. The former have come to be called the *old old* and the latter the *young old*. Because those aged over 90 constitute only a tiny fraction of any even quite numerically large sample of the old old, however, little can be learned about them from such research. Only a study specifically aimed at the 90 and over year olds can throw authentic light on their health and well-being, on what surviving to that great age means to them and what benefits and costs it entails for them and their informal carers. The value of a study, such as the one conducted by Mike Bury and Anthea Holme, of a representative national sample of individuals aged 90 or more, cannot be exaggerated. It is true that subsequent survivors to that great age will not necessarily resemble those studied in this survey in the late 1980s. They will, after all, have had different earlier life experiences which will influence their physical and mental health in old age as well as the meanings, positive and negative, they attach to the feat of surviving so much longer than most of their own contemporaries. Nevertheless, greater knowledge of the life circumstances of today's nonagenarians and centenarians can provide a bench mark against which to observe future generations of survivors. In short, some systematic knowledge, particularly if it is contextualized, as it has been in the study recorded here, is better than the virtually complete ignorance which has existed until now.

Finally, having been associated with the study in an advisory capacity from its beginning to its end, I would like to pay tribute to the two authors for their courage and persistence in meeting and overcoming a range of obstacles which seemed to have been set by the devil to deter them from executing their plans and completing the enterprise.

It is worth reminding readers of some of the problems associated with the kind of survey reported here. In the first place, it proved extremely difficult and laborious to identify the populations aged 90 and over in the various districts randomly selected – a necessary process before selecting, again randomly, a sample of individuals to interview. This preliminary stage alone involved gaining the confidence of and working with the personnel of the National Health Service, local government and voluntary organizations, as well as with the local press and radio. The result of careful work at this stage is an account of the lives of a very representative sample of those aged 90 and over – not the reminiscences of those selected by younger people who are either proud of them or anxious to depict them as intolerable burdens.

Subsequent stages meant recruiting and training interviewers with the ability to undertake work which was undoubtedly more exacting than the general run of survey interviewing, since considerable numbers of the sample had hearing or sight difficulties or were easily fatigued; and relatives and carers, not unnaturally, were anxious to protect the vulnerable and had to be convinced of the researchers' bona fides.

As if these difficulties were not enough, both authors had to cope, at some time during the project, with a serious problem affecting either their own or their family's health. It says much for their dedication and prodigious efforts that they were able to overcome the obstacles and provide such an important contribution to our understanding of the oldest old

Margot Jefferys

ACKNOWLEDGEMENTS

We should like to thank the members of the Charitable Trust which has funded our study, not only for their financial support, but also for the freedom allowed us during the three-and-a-half years of the work.

The study was undertaken on the initiative of the Research Unit of the Royal College of Physicians whose chairman at the time, Sir Cyril Clarke, approached the Department of Social Policy and Social Science, Royal Holloway and Bedford New College. The members of our Advisory Committee were drawn from these two institutions and we should like to thank them all most warmly for their support. We are especially grateful to the chairman, Sir Cyril Clarke, whose unwavering patience and understanding of our problems, advice and specialist knowledge, have been of great value to us throughout the project.

We should particularly like to express our gratitude to Margot Jefferys who has been a source of support to us from the very first. She has provided us throughout with much-needed help and encouragement. Her constructive and critical comments on the book during its preparation have both kept us on our toes and improved the final product considerably. It is, however, only fair to point out that the authors alone carry responsibility for any weaknesses or errors in the text.

There would have been no study without the participation of the individuals aged 90 and over who gave so unstintingly of their time and their thoughts; we thank them most sincerely. We are very grateful also to those representatives of the various services in the eight study areas – too numerous to name individually – who agreed to co-operate, and who gave us much helpful advice and practical help; we drew heavily on their time and their expert knowledge of the field.

We also owe a great debt of gratitude to many other individuals – the list again is too long to thank them all by name – for the advice they gave us at the various stages throughout the study – in selecting the study areas, devising the questionnaire, establishing a methodology, analysing the data, and for reading certain chapter drafts. In particular, we should like to mention Mary Bolam, John Copeland, Karen Dunnell and other members of the OPCS, Mike Wadsworth and Simon Williams. We would also like to acknowledge help from staff at the Centre for Policy on Ageing Library, especially Helen Moneypenny and Gilly Crosby. And we give special thanks to Laurie Letchford, who provided invaluable help in computing the data with skill and endless patience.

Finally, we should like to thank the members of our research team, Didi Rosen, who helped so efficiently and cheerfully in the office during the early months, our excellent interviewers – Valerie Atherton, ·Adrian Barritt, Margaret Birchall, Lesley Currey, Denise Griffin, Sylvia Hale, Jill Mundy, Elizabeth Newman, Linda Nye, Sue Sergeant, Linda Varley, Audrey Waller, Norma Wilkes – and coders – Pauline Lummas, Alison Pennock and Linda Ward. But, above all, our thanks go to Pat Hunt, who provided us with highly skilled and unflagging secretarial support. But more valuable even than this, was her understanding of the work of the project, and her interest in it, which led to an exceptionally close involvement.

LIST OF ABBREVIATIONS
AND NOTE ON NAMES

ADL	Activities of daily living
ADSS	Association of Directors of Social Services
BSG	British Society of Gerontology
CPA	Centre for Policy on Ageing
CSO	Central Statistical Office
DMEC	District Medical Ethical Committee
DHSS	Department of Health and Social Security
DOE	Department of the Environment
FPC	Family Practitioner Committee
GHS	General Household Survey
GP	General Practitioner
HMSO	Her Majesty's Stationery Office
LMC	Local Medical Committee
LSE	London School of Economics
MMF	Millbank Memorial Fund
NCCOP	National Committee for the Care of Old People
NALGO	National Association of Local Government Officers
NHS	National Health Service
NHSCR	National Health Service Central Register
NISW	National Institute for Social Work
OPCS	Office of Population Censuses and Surveys
PDS	Percentage Disability Score
PPS	Probability proportionate to size
PSI	Policy Studies Institute
QALYS	Quality-of-life adjusted years
SPSSx	Statistical Package for the Social Sciences
WHO	World Health Organization

NOTE ON NAMES

All the sample members have been given fictitious names; they have not been identified as belonging to any of the eight named areas of the study.

INTRODUCTION

This book is about the experience of very old age in England today. It is about people who were born in the last twenty years of the nineteenth century and are the survivors of their generation. In future, there are likely to be more survivors from subsequent cohorts. We cannot say with any certainty if life after 90 will be the same or different for them, if only because future survivors will have come from a different generational and social background. The present book, however, is an attempt to offer the beginnings – a bench mark, perhaps – for a better understanding of very old age, and for further research.

BACKGROUND AND AIMS

There have always been old people in society but never before have their numbers and proportions been as large as we find today in most of the developed nations. This is especially true of the very old. The population aged 85 and over in England and Wales, for example, has been growing at 3.8 per cent per annum throughout the 1980s, an 'exceptional' rate of population growth (Warnes 1989: 60). More dramatic is the projected increase for those aged 90 and over, for whom the estimate of 146,423 in 1981 (OPCS 1983a: Table 2), including approximately 2,500 centenarians (Thatcher 1981), is projected to rise to an estimated 231,000 in 1991 (OPCS 1985a: Table 1) and to over 300,000 by the end of the decade (ibid.). Such an increase, numerically and as a proportion of all elderly people, in itself affects the way they are perceived.

Long life, including, particularly, the factors which might promote it, is of perennial interest to human beings, but the circumstances of very old people less so. The reality of very old age is remote from young people, and many middle-aged and even 'young elderly' adults regard it with feelings of considerable ambivalence. Whilst there is

1

much discussion about ageing in today's society, there is less willingness to examine the assumptions which underpin our attitudes towards old age, especially very old age. These assumptions are based on a variety of contradictory positive and negative sentiments, which coalesce into stereotypes.

As part of the positive stereotype, survival into the tenth decade, and even more so to the age of 100 and beyond, is a sign of success and achievement. To be 100 'not out' is to have passed a special, even magical, number. Because of its rarity it takes on exceptional meaning, warranting entry in the record books, notice perhaps by the media and, in Britain, a likely telegram of congratulations from the Queen.

The apparent 'denial of death', which very old people, and centenarians, in particular, represent, acts as a powerful image of the triumph of life over adversity. The presence of very old people in society offers reassurance that, although death cannot be postponed for ever, 'premature death' is not inevitable. Very old people are often described as 'wonderful', 'remarkable', 'amazing' and so on. The languages of admiration and disbelief intermingle, expressing the conscious and unconscious perceptions of survival held by younger people. Moreover, perceptions of very long life are often coloured by the belief that old people were accorded more respect and had more authority in the past, and that this may still be the case in 'simpler' societies. Although this view is open to question (Fennell et al. 1988), it remains a powerful image in popular thought.

Popular negative views of very old age, provide a darker side to the picture. Though death may be denied, it cannot be far away. Very old people remind us of the imminence of death rather than of its postponement. Pity supersedes admiration, and from being thought wonderful, very old people cause distress, are seen as depressing and even threatening. Closely associated with these attitudes is the question of physical and mental decline, and the spectre of dependency. Helplessness and senility are seen to be the epitome of the last phase of the life course.

We might also note here that the negative stereotyping of very old age is not confined to the patronizing or thoughtless young. Even those fully committed to a positive view of ageing, who have done so much to forward this approach, tend to allow this to fall short of extreme old age. Norman (1980: 10), for example, writes of the coming 'explosion [our italics] of the numbers suffering from chronic brain failure' as a consequence of increasing numbers of very old people, without clear evidence that such consequences are inevitable. And Laslett (1987), in outlining his perspective of the life course based on four social ages, whilst effectively challenging the self-evident nature of chronogical age, also stops short where the oldest old are concerned. Membership of the 'Third Age' seems to be offered to the 'middle-aged' who have ceased employment and the active 'young elderly'. The 'Fourth Age' is explicitly placed chronologically at the end of the line and is characterized largely by 'decline and decrepitude'. Laslett (1989) has recently sought to reject this interpretation of his view of the third and fourth ages, though it remains open to argument.

Other perspectives on 'the ageing population' reveal similar difficulties. Arguments, for example, about changes in the pattern of human survival and the production of what has been called a 'rectangular' survival curve, form part of a generally positive view of improvements in longevity and the future for elderly persons, but remain ambiguous as far as the very old are concerned (Bury 1988). The main idea behind the 'rectangularization' argument is that, throughout the twentieth century, an increasing proportion of the population has reached the limits of the 'natural lifespan', largely as the result of the near elimination of 'premature death' (Fries 1980: 132). This improved mortality produces an increasingly rectangularized survival curve, as illustrated in Figure I.1.

Brody (1985), for example, estimates that for the US 'within a very few years about half the population will live more than eighty years'. Similar trends can be observed in Britain. Jefferys (1990) has recently pointed out that 'over half the males born in the 1980s can expect to survive until well beyond their seventieth birthday, and their female counterparts to nearer their eightieth'. Whilst the ideal rectangular survival curve will never be fully realized, an increasing proportion of the population will come near to it.

If, in addition, morbidity (illness and disability) can be 'compressed' into the last years, if not months, of life, the prospect for a vigorous old age is enhanced. 'Postponement of chronic illness thus results in a rectangularization not only of the mortality curve but also of the morbidity curve' (Fries 1980: 133). From this viewpoint, longevity is accompanied by improvement in health and the quality of life. Fries's view, however, is based on the presumption that the 'natural lifespan' is fixed, limiting the period of final illness and decline, and, indeed, the numbers of the very old. So, we again find that a positive outlook on old age as a whole is linked to a view of very old age as either marginal, or characterized by decline and death.

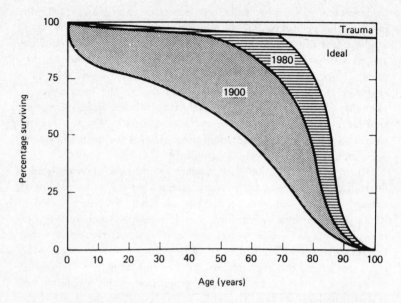

Figure I.1 The increasingly rectangular survival curve
Source: Fries (1980)

All these interpretations, positive as well as negative, need to be exposed to empirical evidence. Without such evidence, the re-drawing of the boundaries between age groups and the focusing of attention on very old age may simply shift the presumed 'burden' of old age onto a newly constructed grouping. The idea, for instance, that very old age is characterized by extreme frailty and dependence relies on two observations based on secondary aggregate data.

First, is the rise with age in the prevalence of chronic illness, disability and dementia (Wells 1979; Martin *et al.* 1988) and second is the general increase with age in the use of health and social services (OPCS 1989: Fig.12h), and the proportion of public spending devoted to elderly people, even though the manner in which these costs are estimated makes them little more than 'guestimates' (Maynard 1989: 49, 50). The problem is that such data may mask wide variations *within* particular age groups, including the very old. There is also a need to recognize that an assumption of worsening health with age takes no account of the changing expectations and values placed on different kinds of activities and health states across the life course. On the second point, there is continuing debate about the possible under-use as well as

4

the over-use of the health and social services (see e.g. Ford and Taylor 1985; Freer 1988). Similarly, high levels of expenditure may disguise the fact that they arise from a variety of different needs and problems.

It is within this context of contradictory views that we formulated our research questions, with the basic objective of providing first-hand evidence to be derived from interviews with very old people themselves. Much discussion of old age is based on data collected through surveys of the general population, which divide the elderly into chronological groupings frequently covering twenty or thirty years of life. There was a need, we felt, for a more focused study of specific age groups within the elderly population, particularly of very old people, in order to test the assumptions which are becoming more prevalent about their state of health and social circumstances. It was necessary, then, to define what we meant by very old age.

In Britain, people receiving the statutory pension (at ages 65 for men and 60 for women) are usually categorized in statistics as elderly, but this is more an administrative device than a meaningful social category. Problems of definition become even more difficult in considering 'the oldest old', a term which has been employed in recent debate, but has not been closely defined (see e.g. *MMF Quarterly* 1985). Oldest old can mean 75 plus, 80 plus, 90 plus or even 100 plus.

For our purposes, centenarians would have been too limited in scope and numbers.The problem of defining the oldest old as those aged 75 and over, or even 80 and over, is that they would still cover a possible span of up to twenty or thirty years and, as previous studies of people in these age groups have shown, the great majority have inevitably been below the age of 90, with the result that those above this age have been neglected. If we wish to find out more about those aged 90 and over, particularly in the light of their increasing numbers, we need to concentrate on them as a group. Moreover, by taking those aged 90 and over, we could be sure that we were focusing attention on the survivors of a specific generation.

We started the study with three main aims. First, we wished to discover what the quality of life was like for people aged 90 and over. Problematic though this concept is, we wished to explore what we took to be its various components, notably, health status, material circumstances, 'morale' and well-being and the extent and character of the support and care very old people receive. We set out to cover all possible residential settings in the community and in communal establishments, and, most importantly, we wanted to obtain the information – both about circumstances and responses to them – as far as possible from the elderly people themselves by means of self-reports.

Secondly, we hoped to explore further the meanings underlying the concept of the quality of life in very old age by investigating the relationship between subjective views and objective circumstances. At the individual level, this meant bringing into the picture the past as well as the present; the experience of historical events, such as wars and economic upheavals, as well as personal ones, such as the age of leaving school and occupational history, though these latter are partly defined by features of changing social structures.

Thirdly, we hoped that our attempts to provide an assessment of the quality of life would be of value to those engaged in planning and implementing policies for very old people.

We based these aims on the assumption that very old age is a social as well as a biological phenomenon, characterized by social patterning and diversity, especially in relation to gender and place of residence, and that this social patterning has come about in response to historical circumstances and biographical experiences over an exceptionally long life course, providing a sense of generation as well as age. This sense of unique generation, of difference, then had to be considered in relation to interdependence with other groups – age-related, occupational, familial – across the life course and in the present.

This social perspective, as distinct from that based on biological and physiological changes alone, would, we hoped, challenge currently held values attached to the outcome of the ageing process, particularly the view that physical and mental frailty and overwhelming dependency are inevitable features of life after 90.

There was a fourth and subsidiary aim concerning the issue of longevity itself. We hoped to identify some of the possible influences – biological, social and cultural, that are associated with survival into the tenth decade and beyond.

Setting out to study very old age in this way also involved a methodological assumption, namely, that it would be possible to identify and interview enough people aged 90 and over to allow us to draw conclusions about the lives of the 90-plus population as a whole.

The chapters that follow will show how far we were able to realise our aims.

SCHEME OF THE BOOK

The first two chapters introduce the study. Chapter 1 describes the way in which we set about the research – our methodology. Chapter 2 then

6

outlines the basic characteristics of the sample members, including their past experiences of education and work, as well as their current living arrangements and material circumstances. In Chapter 3 we go on to explore some of the main influences on longevity among this age group. In Chapter 4 we discuss the crucial issue of health in very old age and present our findings on such matters as chronic illness, disability and mental health.

Material circumstances and health are clearly important to a consideration of the quality of life at any age. In Chapter 5 we examine the concept of the quality of life more fully, with special reference to very old age. This acts as a bridge to the second half of the book which focuses on subjective aspects of experiencing very old age. In Chapter 6 we explore the quality of everyday life for the very old. In Chapter 7 we discuss the difficult issues of dependency, reciprocity and choice, and in Chapter 8 we consider the subject of social support and care, including the experiences of carers. In all these chapters, where relevant, we discuss the differences for the individual between life in a private household and in a communal establishment. Finally, in Chapter 9 we summarize the findings and discuss the main issues raised in earlier chapters.

1

THE STUDY INTRODUCED

In this chapter we broadly describe how we identified the population of people aged 90 and over, how we found the sample, how we approached the people we wished to interview, the questions we asked and the method of interviewing. Finally, we discuss the general outcome of our methodological approach. Technical details will be found in Appendix 1. We also give there an account of our method of analysing the data.

THE 90–PLUS POPULATION

Selection of the areas

In order to gain a representative sample, it was necessary to give every person aged 90 and over in England an equal chance of being selected. Yet we had to confine our interviewing to defined areas in order to make best use of our resources. Identifying those aged 90 and over is particularly difficult as there are no local statistics available for this age group to work from. To overcome this problem, and with advice from the Office of Population Censuses and Surveys (OPCS), we adopted the method of area selection based on the principle of 'probability proportionate to size' (PPS) (Hedges 1977), using local area data for those aged 80 and over (OPCS 1984). Initially, we aimed to interview in twelve areas, which included two London boroughs (for further details on the method of area selection and the PPS method see Appendix 1, section 1).

We then, however, met two major difficulties in moving forward. The first of these concerned one of the London boroughs where, coincidentally, we were piloting the questionnaire. Some of the professionals and service providers with whom we came into contact were extremely helpful and interested in the research. Others, however, erected insurmountable barriers in our path which forced us to abandon the area.

By this time, we recognized that eight areas was the maximum number that we could handle with limited staff and finances. In order to capitalize on the preparatory work already under way, these were chosen at random from the eleven areas already identified (excluding the abandoned London area). It is these eight areas which form the basis of the study.

Method of identification

Having selected the areas, the next task was to set up the relevant sampling frame. Identifying by name all those aged 90 and over was essential to avoid the risk of counting twice. In order to collect these names, we decided to approach *all* the services and agencies which might be concerned with very old people in their locality, or know about them. These included general practitioners (GPs), family practitioner committees (FPCs), the hospital and community health services, social services, housing departments, private and voluntary residential and nursing homes, voluntary agencies, the church and, where appropriate, the local press and radio.

We chose this method of approach, as data from any single source were either deficient in coverage, or for some other reason inadequate, unavailable or unreliable. GP and FPC lists, for instance, are notoriously inaccurate (see e.g. Bowling *et al.* 1988, 1989). The Department of Health and Social Security (DHSS) were not prepared to allow us to obtain names from records of pensioners; resources did not run to a prior sift of names or addresses from sampling frames such as the Electoral Register or Post Code Address Files.

By seeking saturation coverage, we hoped to discover all the relevant individuals. Moreover, by this means we could hope to minimize the potential obstacle of non-co-operation and gain valuable intermediary contacts. Each area was visited and meetings and discussions were held with representatives of the various services and agencies. This personal contact greatly helped in sorting out problems and establishing the legitimacy of the research.

Even so, compiling lists of named persons continued to present major difficulties. It was not only the DHSS that would not disclose names. We sometimes met resistance from other agencies. Concern about confidentiality has undoubtedly increased in recent years. Some of the medical ethical committees and professional care agencies as well as GPs and administrators, when asked to provide names, refused or were reluctant to do so without the individual's permission. In one or two instances we were unable to overcome the resistance. Where we did so, the assurances required and the committee procedures involved usually caused considerable delays (see Appendix 1, section 2).

In the event, we surmounted the various difficulties of identification and were reasonably confident that we had come close to establishing the total live population of men and women aged 90 years and over living in the eight areas at the time of identification. We also identified a number of people who, it subsequently turned out, were no longer alive. From many of our 'sources' the information provided at the time was, as far as we could tell, reliable. From some, however, which included FPCs, GPs and social services departments, it was often seriously out of date. It seemed to make no difference whether their lists had been compiled by hand or computer; if anything, the latter were worse than the former.

Quite why some GP, and for that matter, FPC lists are an unreliable source of information on their very old patients is something of a puzzle. Exactly where the difficulty lies is hard to establish. The various chains of notification of deaths are clear and, for the most part, mandatory (see Appendix 1, section 3). But somewhere along these chains the links are often weak. The problem appeared often enough to cause concern, and not just from the viewpoint of the present study. Aside from the fact that general practice remuneration is partly based on the age structure of their patient lists, with additional per capita payments for those over 75, the National Health Service Central Register is used for much epidemiological and social research. This makes poor notification especially worrying, though it may be that the failure to keep lists up to date occurred only at *local* level. Whilst we can only report our experience of relatively frequent individual errors discovered in the process of our own identification procedures, we think the problem is significant enough to warrant further attention.

These various notification procedures – obligatory or otherwise – within the health service do not of course apply to the domiciliary social services. Here they must keep their own lists up to date, although this is not always easy. In the present study, as with the health services, we found considerable differences between the study areas in the reliability of the lists. Not surprisingly, information obtained directly from the various residential institutions, statutory or private, was up to date, except, occasionally, from a hospital.

Response to our initial request for names was lower in the case of private residential homes and nursing homes. The proportion of non-replies, varying from area to area, amounted to 30 per cent of the residential homes and 15 per cent of the nursing homes.

Follow-up telephone calls revealed a number of expected reasons – too busy to reply, our letter not received and, most usually, nobody aged 90 and over. Nearly all responded to the follow-up and, among the few who did not, we could discount the risk of losing more than the possible single name, because of coverage from other sources. We were not in a position to investigate the few who remained persistently incommunicado. We cannot say, therefore, if this was an indication of dubious secrecy, a dislike of research on the part of owners and managers or simply a sense of protectiveness towards residents or patients.

Reliability of the identified populations aged 90 plus

Table 1.1 shows the estimated male and female populations in the eight areas. The estimates are from our original identifications. They must, however, be viewed with caution in the light of the later discovery, at the field stage, of the many deaths which had occurred in the identified populations either before or after we had been notified of their existence. Not surprisingly, this age group proved difficult to find as the numbers diminish with every advancing year as a result of high mortality. For the sake of accuracy, using figures that discounted death before identification, we attempted a revision of the estimates (see Appendix 1, section 4). The true picture is probably somewhere between the two estimates, but we have been advised by OPCS to let the original ones stand as the basis of our study.

As is well known, in the older age groups women far exceed men. We were pleased to find, as can be seen in Table 1.2, that the male/female proportions in the present study reflect those of the estimated population aged 90 and over in England and Wales.

Selection and stratification of the sample

We hoped to interview 200 people but clearly could not hope for a 100 per cent response. To allow for a reasonable failure rate, therefore, we selected a target sample of 260 (see Appendix 1, section 5).

Where a sample is small and particularly when it is taken from an elderly population in which there is certainly an imbalance of the sexes,

11

Table 1.1 Total number of men and women aged 90 and over in the eight areas (original estimates)

Area	Women	Men	Total
Broadland	262	74	336
Chichester	751	230	981
Dudley (est)	725	150	875
Maidstone	364	72	436
New Forest	790	225	1,015
Sefton	1,134	221	1,355
S Shropshire	164	42	206
Wear Valley	193	46	239
Total	4,383	1,060	5,443

Table 1.2 The age and sex composition of the identified 90–plus population compared with that of England and Wales

	90-plus population		
	Present study		England and Wales
	as estimated in the eight areas: 1987 %		1986* %
Women			
90–94	61.0	} 80.5	61.6 } 80.0
95+	19.5		18.4
Men			
90–94	14.8	} 19.5	16.6 } 20.0
95+	4.7		3.4
		100	100
Total	(5,443)		

*Source: unpublished OPCS estimates

it is advisable to stratify so as to ensure adequate representation of groups which might be underrepresented in a random sample. We divided our population into four groups: an equal number (65) of each were then selected at random.

In this way, the sample proportions, relative to the 'true' situation, were deliberately skewed in favour of men and the older age groups, so that we should have enough people in these groups to study. To discuss the characteristics as a whole, their health status, attitudes and so on, on the basis of equal or near-equal proportions, however, would give a false impression. In the analysis, therefore, we have, where appropriate, adopted the standard technical device of weighting to redress this imbalance and re-establish the sample as it would have been in its original 'correct' proportions (for the meaning and method of weighting see Appendix 1, section 6).

In subsequent chapters, we have broadly adopted two approaches in referring to the sample data. When we are discussing the sample where it represents members of the total 90–plus population (provided our replies approximate to the total possible number), we use 'weighted' figures. In other words, we have multiplied or divided the actual figures of the sample members to correspond as far as possible to those of the respective age and sex groups in the 90–plus population.

Secondly, when we compare the four main groups of the sample – women aged 90–94 and 95 plus; men aged 90–94 and 95 plus – or describe and comment on the people interviewed, then we are referring to the *actual* sample.

We also found it appropriate to use the actual sample figures when discussing the carers' and the interviewers' assessments. As a result, the percentages given cannot be taken to represent the proportions of 'carers' of people aged 90 and over. They remain, nonetheless, illustrative of important issues.

THE SAMPLE STUDIED

The selected sample

It is, of course, inevitable that among people belonging to the chosen age group there will be some who will die between the date of selection and that of the projected interview. Those of our initial sample who were no longer alive or did not otherwise 'qualify' for inclusion in the study we designated 'out-of-scope' (Morton-Williams 1979), and picked other names from our identified populations to substitute for them. We found, however, that some of the substituted names were of individuals who were also out-of-scope and set about getting substitutes for them too (see Appendix 1, section 5, Table A1.4). In the end, the exercise became unmanageable, especially for the sample of men aged 95 and over in some areas, and we eventually abandoned the search. Our final sample, therefore, namely, those we hoped to interview, included only 222 people rather than our target number of 260. These we designated as 'in-scope'. Seventeen of them were centenarians (see Appendix 1, section 7).

Table 1.3 Response rate by sex and age: selected sample

	Women			Men			Total
	90–94	95+	Total %	90–94	95+	Total %	%
Interviewed	46	47	78.2	54	36	87.4	82.4
Refusals/ denials of access	14	12	21.8	9	4	12.6	17.6
Total	60	59	100 (119)	63	40	100 (103)	100 (222)

The response rate

Table 1.3 shows the response rate of the in-scope sample and how this was distributed between the four age/sex groups. For people of such an advanced age we regarded a response rate of more than 82 per cent as very satisfactory. It was, we think, partly a result of very careful preparation for the interviewing. In fact, it was the women, particularly the 'younger' women, who exercised their right of refusal in greater proportions than the men. In some cases, of course, refusal was not necessarily an individual's choice; family members or other carers might also be involved. Fourteen of the seventeen selected centenarians were interviewed, either directly or by proxy.

Representativeness

We have seen that the identified 90–plus population in the eight areas corresponds broadly to the equivalent national proportions. So, too, after weighting, did the sample interviewed (see Table 1.4).

Other factors, however, must also be taken into account in making an assumption of representativeness, not least, the proportions living at home and in residential accommodation.

An accurate picture of the level of residential, nursing-home and hospital provision for elderly people is still difficult to construct (Challis and Bartlett 1988: 20, 24), partly because the situation is changing very fast and definitions are difficult to arrive at. To obtain national figures for our age group is virtually impossible. It is clear, however, that the percentage of the elderly population in institutional accommodation increases markedly with age. Laing (1988: 237), for

Table 1.4 Subjects interviewed by sex and age: weighted sample

	%	
Women		
90–94	62.0	
		80.0
95+	18.0	
Men		
90–94	17.0	
		20.0
95+	3.0	
Total	100	
	(200)	

instance, suggests that about 15 per cent of the English population aged 85 and over are in residential homes compared with just over 3 per cent of those aged 75 to 84. With such a rapid rate of increase, a considerably greater rise would be expected for those aged 90 and over. For all those aged 85 and over Laing estimates that the proportion in *all* types of establishment has risen to 20 per cent (ibid).

Extrapolating from these trends, it is therefore not surprising to find a considerably higher proportion of people aged 90 and over no longer living in their own homes. The proportion in this category among our selected sample was 47 per cent (87 per cent of whom were interviewed, thereby just reversing the proportions), which is in line with these trends of rapid increase.

We recognize with regret that the absence of a London borough in some degree impairs the full national representativeness of our sample and we do not know with any certainty what effect this exclusion may have. There is no reason to suppose, however, that it affects sex, or other potential sources of bias. We can assert that our sample is likely to be representative of England, excluding Greater London. We are able to present a picture of life based on a wide variety of urban and rural settings and in a diversity of social contexts and circumstances.

THE PILOT STUDY

The pilot exercise was not only important in the design of the questionnaire and the conducting of the interviews, but also gave us invaluable insights into all the preliminary procedures. The difficulties

Table 1.5 Subjects interviewed by sex and age according to type of informant: actual sample

	Women		Men	
	90–94 %	95+ %	90–94 %	95+ %
Subject	65.2	48.9	75.9	66.7
Part proxy	17.4	31.9	14.8	27.8
All proxy	17.4	19.2	9.3	5.5
Total	100	100	100	100
	(46)	(47)	(54)	(36)

encountered in the London borough taught us many lessons useful for our approach elsewhere.

In the second area – Chichester – a mixed urban–rural district in the south of England, the response of the medical, hospital and community health services was excellent. The release of names to us, however, was a sticking point with the Director of Social Services. This area was, in fact, one of the eight later selected for the main study, and the problem was eventually circumvented by goodwill (see Appendix 1, section 10).

THE INTERVIEWS

Proxy interviews

We decided that to obtain information about as many individuals as possible in our sample, we should use proxies if it were absolutely necessary. In the event, as can be seen from Table 1.5, the proportion of subjects for whom we had to use a proxy for the whole interview was relatively small. Among the older men, for instance, this was as low as just over 5 per cent. In a further 28 per cent of interviews with this group a proxy helped. Thus, 67 per cent were solely with the subject, a proportion topped – at 76 per cent – by the male 90–94 age group, reflecting important differences in the health and independence of particular groups in the study, an issue to which we shall return in later chapters.

Sometimes the help of a relative or member of staff was needed to act as 'interpreter'. This might be because of severe deafness, some memory loss or confusion or general frailty. The interviewers' manner of handling these joint interviews varied according to the degree of intervention necessary to get a reply that was as full as possible, yet remained 'uncontaminated' by the proxy's own views. Proxy opinions as opposed to proxy factual accounts of past and present circumstances would be considered invalid though we recognize that the division is not always clear. Joint interviews were often full and satisfactory, unlike those where reliance was entirely on a proxy.

Carer interviews

Carer interviews – 158 in all, 86 per cent of the number of main interviews – were usually arranged at the time of the main interview, and only carried out with the respondent's agreement. The questionnaire was short, the interview usually lasting for about half an hour except where the carer clearly felt a need to talk.

The questions

The main questionnaire was initially designed to allow for the possibility that a proportion of our respondents might have difficulty in sustaining a long interview, and that there might be problems for some in understanding even relatively straightforward questions. Connected with this last point, we also assumed that deafness or problems with comprehension might induce the need to repeat a question, at least in a proportion of our interviews. Re-phrasing might help understanding. So, although the questions, with one exception, were formulated as direct questions demanding a reply, interviewers were allowed to use different wording, provided, of course, that the sense was preserved.

The questionnaire combined structured and semi-structured components. The main exception to the question/answer formula was a request at the beginning of the main central section of the questionnaire that our respondents describe a typical recent day in their lives.

The idea of trying to open up the topic of everyday life, providing little by way of guidance other than prompts, was only partially successful in the aim of motivating a spontaneous response. Bucke and Insley (1976) had used this method successfully in their small study of centenarians. In our study, a few people rattled through their day, with evident pleasure, needing little prompting. With some, the exercise had to be abandoned, and in between was a range of responses calling for greater or less prompting. The results, however, have proved useful in providing illustrations, which we have drawn on in presenting the findings.

17

In designing the study we attempted to strike a balance between a research instrument that would allow us to explore a range of subjective views, yet provide a profile of the sample which would give us the basis for comparing individuals and the different groupings within the sample (for the main areas of questioning see Appendix 1, section 8).

Where possible, as is common practice, we drew on tried – and tested – questions from elsewhere (see Appendix 1, section 9). On the whole, interviewers did not report widespread difficulties as the result of ambiguities or confusion with the questions. We attempted to build in 'validity checks' (de Vaus 1986) on the information gathered from each respondent, by the comparison of 'internal' replies, and by 'external checks' (Oppenheim 1966) through the carer interviews and an additional assessment by the interviewers.

Approach to the individuals

The three main principles of the approach to the people we hoped to interview were first, that they should have adequate warning of our wishes and intentions, secondly, that they should be approached initially by someone they knew (see Appendix 1, section 10), and thirdly, that they or their representatives should be given a fair opportunity to refuse an interview, though, where appropriate, gentle persuasion was not ruled out. We were able to translate these principles into action largely by dint of our established relationship with the various services and agencies who had supplied the names, not one of whom, we are grateful to say, failed to co-operate on this further exercise.

In our view, the fact that the first request for their participation in the research came from someone they knew undoubtedly helped to promote the atmosphere of goodwill in which nearly all the interviews were conducted, as well as encouraging an initially positive response. One male resident in a local authority home was reported by the warden as being 'very aggressive; he nearly blew a fuse when the letter was read to him. Sorry!'. For the most part, however, the refusals or denials of access by relatives or establishment staff came as a tick against the 'no' on the return slips. These were often accompanied by an apologetic little note, just as the acceptances often included a welcoming one.

The interviewers and, where appropriate, one of us, together with the providers of the names, were closely involved in the various follow-up procedures, that is, in arranging interviews with those who had agreed, in recording the refusals, in attempting to trace 'non-existent' people and in finding substitutes for those who had died or who were untraceable.

These were, as can be imagined, busy weeks, for our aim was to conduct the field work simultaneously in all the areas. Interviewers were able to start interviewing while substitute seeking proceeded; the bulk of the interviewing lasted for only eight weeks.

Presentation of the questionnaire

Presentation of the questionnaire is as important as design, particularly with a study group such as ours. Elderly, often frail, people are especially vulnerable to the sins of commission and omission of run-of-the-mill survey techniques. The interviewers were all trained and experienced and, for the most part, familiar with their localities. Intensive briefing and mock interviews had taken place before the field work began.

Use of tape recorders

The questionnaire introduction referred to the intention of tape recording the interview. Experience had shown that an assumption of acceptance of this idea was rewarded with untroubled agreement, whereas a tentative 'would-you-mind' approach resulted quite often in refusal. Only one of the elderly people and one carer raised an objection to the idea, and on two occasions we were asked for a copy of the tape. The main object of recording the interviews was to provide examples to illustrate our conclusions, and to give some life to the bare statistics. Furthermore, listening to the tapes has given us considerable insight into the nature of the response and the personalities of the interviewees, as well as the process of interviewing itself.

The length of the interviews

The staying power of the elderly individuals was on the whole considerable. Other researchers in this field will not be surprised at the fact that if anyone was exhausted by the end of the interview it was the questioner as often as the person questioned.

There were a large number of questions and potentially over 1,000 different items of information for each person which, theoretically, could be used to contrast them with one another. In the pilot study we had found that one and a half hours could normally comfortably accommodate all the relevant questions, with an additional half hour or less for the carer interview. In the main study there was, not unexpectedly, considerable variation, the longest interview lasting four hours and the shortest, twenty-five minutes. But the average interview did in fact last one and a half hours, and there were very few complaints about the length of time or indeed about any other aspect of the interview.

THE RESULTS

The results of the survey will, of course, prove to be the test of our methodology (for the method of analysis see Appendix 1, section 11). A preoccupation with methodology, however, can sometimes mean having to search for a substance. Indeed, it has been our experience that method and substance are often more closely aligned than is sometimes recognized.

In the first place, the desire to establish a *representative* sample of people aged 90 years and over, created many headaches for us, which reflected real problems in the field as well as self-imposed technical hurdles. The difficulties, for example, that we encountered in identifying individuals aged 90 years and over, both from national statistics and from local sources, often reinforced our feelings that the very old are indeed treated as members of a residual category. No doubt, official records of people of all ages are 'inaccurate' in many ways (and there are reasons to be thankful that this is the case). But, during the identification stage, on finding that people who were thought to be alive had, in fact, been dead for many years, we constantly asked ourselves what did this mean for those who *were* alive?

Moreover, the quantity of letter writing (something in excess of 2,000 letters) that was necessary in order to gain access to our subjects, as well as highlighting the afore-mentioned problem, also revealed aspects of protectiveness towards the very old that warrant further examination. Much of the time we fully understood the concern of agencies, establishments and family members for the welfare of the individual in question. But we were not convinced that this was always the central issue. The rights of the elderly and the very old to make choices and exercise control over their own lives are as important as for any other group of adults. We are, of course, aware of the dependence of many elderly people and their vulnerability to exploitation, but these issues should not be used as an impenetrable shield against the outside world as a whole. Our experience suggests that there is often a fine line between legitimate protectiveness and overprotection.

Finally, in spite of the difficulties we encountered in establishing a 'typical day', the process of interviewing itself disclosed important features of the daily life of our respondents. The main problems in interviewing centred inevitably on the frailty - physical and mental - of some of the respondents. Dementia or severe confusion were in one sense easier to cope with than partial confusion or memory loss, since the former was usually known about beforehand and appropriate proxy arrangements could be made. The most obvious difficulty concerned deafness. In reading and listening to the interviewers' comments after the event, and even more so in listening to the interviews on tape, we were made painfully aware of the problems of communication brought about by hearing difficulties.

In short, our identification, sampling and interviewing procedures involved both technical and substantive issues throughout the months of the survey. Generally, the findings of this study confirmed those of others (e.g. Bucke and Insley 1976; Ridley *et al.* 1979) that it is possible to obtain reliable information from very old people.

2

THE PEOPLE INTRODUCED

Whatever we may feel about the assignment of very old people to a residual, or marginal status, or about the notice afforded them as a 'burden' or, in contrast, as an elite, the fact remains that, viewed historically, the span of their ninety or more years places them in a category apart. Nowhere is this more apparent than in their past and present circumstances, aspects of which we now consider.

Many of these circumstances have implications for the issue of longevity, or for the quality of their lives. These we discuss in later chapters; here we present the simple picture. We look at the proportions of women and men aged 90 and over; their marital status; their education and employment history including retirement; the impact on their lives of war and economic upheaval; their social class; their financial circumstances; particulars of their residence and their living arrangements. We illustrate the discussion with our survey data and individual examples from the study.

SEX AND MARITAL STATUS

It is a well-known fact, confirmed by our findings as shown in Chapter 1, that there is an enormous preponderance of women among the oldest members of the population. A ratio of four women to one man gives us the first characteristic of the age group which distinguishes it from others.

The various possible causes of this imbalance of the sexes, reflecting historical circumstances, most notably the impact of war and disease and the chances of survival for men into later life in the twentieth century, are important for the issue of longevity, which we discuss in Chapter 3.

Table 2.1 Marital status by sex: weighted sample

Marital status	Women %	Men %
Single	13.8	7.5
Married	3.1	22.5
Widowed	83.1	70.0
Total	100	100
	(160)	(40)

The second factor common to people aged 90 and over to a far greater extent than to any other age group, even the immediately preceding one, has to do with marital status. If a woman has been married and has reached the age of 90 or more, the estimated chances of being a widow are about eighteen to one (OPCS 1983a: Table 6). As can be seen in Table 2.1, the chances among our female sample were even higher (only two women in the actual sample, both in the younger age group, still had husbands living).

We may pause to reflect what such widespread widowhood entails, but in doing so should also note that, as likely as not, it is long-standing. Most of the sample had lost their spouses many years previously, particularly the women, for whom the average period was twenty-nine years. Some women, therefore, will have been widowed for as long as they had been married, or longer. This is something we shall be looking at again in Chapter 6, since the effects of bereavement must depend to some extent on how recently it has occurred.

Not all the married men (among whom three were aged between 95 and 100) were living at home with their wives. The average length of bereavement among the men, not surprisingly, was less than for the women – fifteen years – and they had made twice as many second marriages. Mr Bickerton was one. He had remarried at the age of 87. Now aged 90, he was living with his 76-year-old wife.

Also reflecting persistent sex differences are the proportions of single women and men among the very old, estimated nationally at 16 per cent and 8 per cent respectively (ibid); 14 per cent and 8 per cent respectively among our sample.

It is not, however, only present circumstances which distinguish very old people as a group from others. We found such distinctions in some of the earlier circumstances of their lives, not least their education history.

EDUCATION

Age of leaving school

Today secondary education begins at the age of 11 or, for those in the private system, at 13 or 14. It must not end before the age of 16. Even at that age it is now official policy to retain all those who are not able to get jobs in some form of education or training. But circumstances were different in the first decade of this century when most members of our sample would have reached the present secondary school age. The 1870 Education Act was concerned with elementary education and, although the 1902 Act introduced a state system of *secondary* education, it was not until 1907 that its provision began to have any meaning for the population as a whole.

Only a minority of our sample, marginally more men than women, were able to take advantage of any opportunities for non-state secondary education, (see Appendix 2, Table A2.1), reflecting the situation in the nation at large. Mrs Forbes was one of the women who did. A 96-year-old widow whose father and husband had both been solicitors, now living in a private rest home, she described a fairly typical life of an upper-class young woman of the period:

> I left school at 18 and then went to 'finish' in France. I could only stay for six months as my mother became ill and, as there were five of us, I had to return to run the house and servants.

As many as 75 per cent of the women and 72 per cent of the men had left school at the age of 13 or 14 or even earlier. Mr Baldwin, for instance, had left at 'about 9': 'I went to school in London, down Sloane Square. We had to pay twopence a week and take our pens and pencils with us.'

At least twenty-one members of the actual sample remembered 11 as the age at which they left school. Mr Sadler recalled clearly his post-school 'childhood': 'I worked on farms in the summer and made hoops for barrels in winter. I earned eightpence a day.'

Ninety-three-year-old Miss Spencer and 90-year-old Mrs Horden both left school at the age of 13. The former learned shorthand and typing afterwards, and worked in the same insurance firm for thirty-six years. Mrs Horden was one of the few members of the sample who described themselves as 'delicate' in childhood. She had, apparently, spent 'more time at home than in my convent school'.

The pattern of minimal education for the majority is clear. It is a pattern that distinguishes nonagenarians and centenarians from the young and middle-aged in particular. It was not until 1944 that universal secondary education reached the statute books and the school leaving age was raised to 15, though, as the century advanced, so more and more people did in fact stay on at school, if only for an extra year or two.

Further education

Leaving school at a comparatively early age did not, as we have already seen in Miss Spencer's case, necessarily mean the end of their education. But relatively few women in the sample had had any formal further education. Mrs Hopkins, 95 years old, the daughter of a shipper and the widow of a chartered accountant, was another exception. She went on to Manchester University, eventually becoming an infant teacher – 'I loved it'. Among the men something over one-quarter had had some kind of part-time education, and a further small minority full-time.

The consequent dearth of qualifications is no surprise. Miss Hill, an ex-headmistress, qualified in English and history at Girton College, Cambridge and was awarded a titular degree, a telling marker of life-course differences, since Cambridge degrees proper were not awarded to women until 1948. The subjects for which degrees or an equivalent qualification were obtained by seven men of the actual sample ranged from physics to architecture. A further three from each sex were qualified at a higher education level below that of a degree. Otherwise there was for a handful of the women and some few more of the men an assortment of clerical, secretarial, apprenticeship, trade and similar certificates. Several people referred to self-education.

Set within the framework of their life course, an analogous pattern of experience may be found when we turn to the next major event of their lives – work.

WORKING LIVES

Occupations

Looking back to the early part of this century, we should expect to find considerable differences in the field of employment; no computer programmers or television presenters in those days, no lead miners or tin-plate workers in these. But perhaps the greatest shift which was already just beginning after the First World War, and which gathered momentum after the Second, was from agriculture and heavy industry to light industry and the service industries, the historical shift from manual work to non-manual. Halsey (1986) notes, for example, that in 1911 the labour force was divided three-quarters to a quarter between manual and non-manual groups, respectively. By 1981 female participation in the labour force had grown considerably, three-fifths of which were, by this time, non-manual workers, despite the earlier counter-movement from domestic service into the manufacturing industries.

Should we therefore expect to find a corresponding preponderance of the former group of manual occupations among our sample and their equivalents in the 90–plus population at large? The answer, for two main reasons, is a guarded no. First, many jobs in heavy industry were killers, either directly or indirectly. Coal miners, for instance, have had much higher death rates than men from professional backgrounds (see note 1).

Secondly, the employment histories of some of the men of this generation are likely to have followed the shift in employment patterns. Certainly this was evident among our sample. Two-fifths had had more than one occupation. There was, as would be expected for the earlier part of their working lives, much work with horses and on farms.

Memories of pay – or the lack of it – were often still fresh. Mr Morgan, for instance, described how, as a shop assistant, he was paid £60 a year, of which five shillings a week went for lodgings. Before that he had been apprenticed at a general stores for four years without any pay, ' "living in" they called it'.

Readers of *Akenfield* will recall the hardships of life in a Suffolk village at the turn of the century: 'we dreaded the rain; it washed our few shillings away' (Blythe 1969: 48). There were no guaranteed earnings in those days and, what is more, there was the imposition of fines for such 'sins' as lateness. There were no paid holidays, no five-day weeks and the hours were very long. It was a very different picture from that of most of present-day Britain or, indeed, of the Britain of twenty or thirty years ago, when the men we are concerned with were coming to the end of their working lives.

There have, too, been great changes in the employment patterns of women. Those from the middle and upper classes at that time were less likely than those of their equivalents of later generations to have been in paid employment at all and, with a few exceptions, this was reflected in the employment histories of our sample of women. Moreover, for all women, there was a more limited range of occupations available and it will come as no surprise that domestic service figured prominently among the reported occupations. Also to be found were those of shop assistant, children's nurse, factory hand, clerk or secretary.

It seems that a substantial majority of the younger women were in paid employment at some period of their lives, nearly all these starting as soon as they left school. Furthermore, judging from the duration of their jobs, at least one-third of this 'employed' group must, like Mrs Benson, have worked right through to the age of retirement. She worked in a jelly-and-custard factory all her life. Mrs Fawcett was another and, as a farmer's wife, recalled with delight her early experiences.

The first farm we were at we had a jolly good cow and I didn't know how to make butter. Anyhow I thought if somebody else can do it, I can do it. That's the attitude you know. I used to make fifteen to sixteen pounds of butter from one cow per week – it was marvellous. I was proud, you know, of course I was proud. I'd not been used to living like that you see.

There were many more full-time housewives among the older than among the younger women but over one-third had been in paid employment, Mrs Vernon, for instance, for forty-six years as an owner of a jewellery shop and Mrs McDonald for fifty years as a 'domestic servant with gentlefolk'.

Of the eleven single women, nine were in paid employment for various lengths of time, five at least for all their working lives.

Miss Moore, now confused and in hospital, had previously lived on her own. Her working life – as a shop assistant – had suffered the fate of many of her single status and generation; her 'duty' took her home to look after her father and an invalid brother after her mother died, a 'carer' in her own time. Miss Gregory, aged 92, had experienced in her past life altogether different circumstances from the other single women of our sample. She had left school at 19, the daughter of an industrialist. With her sister she had adopted two girls, one at nine months and the other at five months, 'I enjoyed that'. At the time of the interview she was living in a large Victorian house with a housekeeper and nurses on six-hour shifts. She ran the house herself, helped by the adopted daughters who visited every week.

Interruptions – wars and the Depression

An account of the working lives of people now aged 90 and over would be incomplete without reference to the major disruption to those working lives, in the shape of the First World War. It was probably the single most formative experience for the men and women of this generation, which is the last to have lived through it as adults. A few of the men in our sample had joined up – 'changed their sky' (Blythe 1969: 37) – before 1914 but the vivid, often poignant or horrific reminiscences were of the war years. Mr Walker, for example, talked of his time in France:

> I was in the Artillery and I was going to the ammunition room carting ammunition with the wagon to the gun lines, and, I don't like to tell you this, but when you advance, going forward, the sergeant major would shout (I can see him now; of course he had his chin strap): 'Now dismount and get your trenching tool and get a shovel full of anything you can see and dig in and throw it over their mouths.' The burial party was in arrears and they are coming up after you digging holes and throwing them in anyway they can – they had to be buried properly later on.
>
> I looked after the horses – they were good horses, poor things, but of course they didn't get enough to eat. We didn't get a lot to eat either – one biscuit – one dog biscuit a day. Nothing to eat and dead hungry. By gow, it was a beggar, honest to God it was that.

Mr Baldwin was one of those 'coming after, digging holes'. Mr Morgan, the unpaid apprentice, also 'drove the guns in the Royal Field Artillery at the age of 19'. He was wounded in 1917 and spent nine months in hospital.

Mr Godwin saw service in the Middle East, joining up in 1914 at the age of 18, and recalled a post-war experience.

> At the reunion in London when the London troops had a march through and I went up to represent my batallion there was only three of us there and we were all out of work and there was all this ceremony going on. And we felt right out of it.

As we all know, the impact of the First World War, with its devastating toll of young male lives, had a different, no less devastating, effect on the women – the loss of husbands, sweethearts, brothers and a future, for many, of enforced spinsterhood. Mrs Forbes, whom we met earlier, was unusual for her generation in that she herself saw war service abroad as well as suffering the sadly more usual bereavement.

I lost a husband in the first war and a son in the second. I married at 23 and had only had six weeks of marriage. We had one weekend together and he was killed at Gallipoli at 23. After, I went out to France to work in the canteen at Calais.

In the Second World War Mrs Forbes drove her car in London for the 'car testers'. She was clearly an enterprising person, as in 1957, at the age of 65, after her second husband died, she went travelling – 'I went off all by myself to Japan, China, Singapore, Hong Kong. People thought I was mad but I loved it. I made such marvellous friends.'

In between the two world wars, Britain saw a period of economic decline and severe unemployment. The Depression was recalled as a 'past event' by some, but more often as an experience to be deplored in general rather than as affecting them personally. Mr Anderson, for instance, recalled that 'you could hardly get into the street with all the people. It was the unemployment, just after the [14 – 18] war, you know.' The period following the Second World War was one of reconstitution and economic development and, by the end of the 1960s, the members of our age group were moving into retirement at a time when full employment was buoyant.

RETIREMENT

For people aged 90 and over, men as well as women, retirement is a matter of past history and, for the great majority, any traumas attaching to the giving up of paid employment are likely to be long since over. As might be expected of employment patterns during this period, most of the male members of the sample retired between the ages of 65 and 70. There were, however, some late retirers. Dr Carey, aged 92, had never officially retired as a GP, was still, he told the interviewer, entitled to sign a death certificate and still had relevant legal powers. Mr Unwin had practised as a pharmacist until he was 80: 'I thought I'd better give it up before I made some stupid mistake which you can't afford to do in that job.'

Three of the men, however, withheld such qualms until a much later age. Mr Spinner, aged 90, still very active had been a chef and retired when he was 86. Mr Dean, aged 97, had spent the first forty-three years of his adult life in the Royal Navy and the last twenty-seven as owner of a grocery and hardware shop from which he retired at the age of 92. He was now in a residential home. Ninety-eight-year-old Mr Foot had been a schoolmaster teaching physics and maths for sixty-one years and had then coached backward children and boys from overseas until 1981 when he was 93. He now lived, very independently and contentedly, with his daughter and her partner.

A few people were still actively engaged in voluntary work, like Mr Godwin and Mr Roberts who were secretaries of their local British Legion branches. These few examples tell us more, perhaps, about professional, skilled or self-employed occupations among survivors than about late or early retirement as a generational characteristic. Indeed, all that we have been discussing concerning employment has, of course, a close relationship with social-class position.

SOCIAL CLASS

Where there had been more than one occupation which was, as we have seen, the case for some numbers of male sample members, these for the most part belonged to the same social-class category, but in a few cases there were indications of upward mobility. This may furthermore be deduced from the early age of school leaving of so many of the sample. For the purposes of assigning the respondents to a Registrar-General's classification category we took the occupation of longest duration.

We have also, in order to assess the social-class position of the sample women, followed the traditional, if unsatisfactory, practice of using spouse's or, where necessary, father's occupation. Table 2.2 shows the social class membership of the total sample.

The picture, with its relatively low proportions of people in classes IV and V, and high ones in classes I and II, carries with it important implications for survival, which we take up in Chapter 3. Here we note only that, though the edges are blurred, there are again some markers which distinguish very old from younger people.

FINANCIAL CIRCUMSTANCES

It is generally held to be the case that the economic and social position of a person in retirement is an extension of his or her earlier position in the labour market (see e.g. Walker 1981, 1983). We look further at this argument in Chapter 7. Meanwhile, the evidence from our sample has some bearing on it. There was a significant association between social class and assumed income level. We have used the qualification 'assumed' because we asked the sample members only for the sources of their income; from this we could do no more than guess at its level. Furthermore, where the elderly individuals were living with relatives,

Table 2.2 The social class membership of men and women using Registrar-General's classification: weighted sample

	Social class	%	%
I	Professional, etc.	15.0	
II	Intermediate	20.3	35.3
III.1	Skilled non-manual	9.1	
III.2	Skilled manual	34.2	43.3
IV	Partly skilled	11.2	
V	Unskilled	5.3	16.5
	Unclassified, including armed services		4.9
			100
			(187)

we did not ascertain the relatives' financial position; equally, for those in establishments, where these were private, we discovered neither the costs nor the extent, if any, of subsidy to the individuals in question.

With the wealth of other material we were attempting to gather from our sample members, the seeking of detailed financial information was not within the scope of the study. Material circumstances must, of course, figure in any assessment of the quality of life. We are, however, primarily concerned with how the elderly people felt about their financial position, and it is in this light that such evidence as we present should be viewed.

Table 2.3 shows the sources of income for the sample as a whole as reported to the interviewers. The majority of the sample members could rely on more than one source of income, reporting, as well as the retirement pension, an occupational pension, savings, or investments singly or in various combinations. On the other hand, as many as 42 per cent depended solely on their statutory retirement pension, with or without the addition of other statutory benefits. Even if there is no rent or mortgage to pay, nobody could claim that such a financial position spells affluence.

Well over half this group were living in communal establishments, and it is important to note that there was generally among those in an institutional setting a significantly lower level of income as measured by its source. Of those solely in receipt of the statutory pension who were living in private households, 30 per cent were sharing a home

Table 2.3 Sources of income: weighted sample

Sources of income	Subjects %
Combined sources: stat. retirement pension, occupational pension; savings; investments, etc.	58.3
Stat. retirement pension only or together with supplementary benefit* and/or other statutory allowances	41.7
	100
	(158)

*Since April 1988 known as income support.

with their children or other relatives. It might thus be assumed that income also, in one way or another, would be shared, even when they were the principal householder (i.e. the home owner or nominated tenant), which was the case for over two-thirds.

The suggestion of poverty amongst a few sample members could be deduced from replies to a question put to them on whether or not they felt they had enough money for their creature comforts. Thirteen per cent felt they had only just enough. Nine members of the actual sample (just under 10 per cent of the total sample) felt themselves to be in financial difficulties; seven of these came from social classes IV and V and seven were dependent solely on their retirement pension, with or without supplementary benefit (now income support) or an additional statutory allowance. Of the total sample, 71 per cent felt they had enough money, and 7 per cent 'more than enough'. These last two groups comprised people from all social classes deriving their incomes from a variety of sources.

Other breakdowns failed to yield any obvious groupings. Of the nine sample members in financial difficulties, for instance, three were in private households, two, as householders on their own; three were in local authority homes, one in a private nursing home; one, Mrs Ellis – against her will, as we shall see in Chapter 7 – in a cottage hospital.

Caution, of course, should be exercised concerning the face value of replies to questions such as these on the adequacy of their income. It is true that a few did signal financial problems. For the majority, the wish not to complain has to be set against the possible development of low expectations with age and the possibility of unmet need and poverty, although as such this did not appear to be widespread.

One of the clichés about elderly people is that as they grow older their material needs diminish. It may be, however, that diminishing need is a reflection of the lack of resources. From our evidence, there appears to be some truth in both points of view. As many as 59 per cent of our elderly people, for example, never went out of doors. Discounting for the moment the reasons for this, it must mean less wear and tear on outdoor clothes and little need for expenditure on transport and outside entertainment. Of those few who said they did have to go without things, clothes were mentioned by only three. Mr Spinner, living alone, said that he did not have enough food, but most usually it was the 'extras' – presents and the like, or Mr Walker's extra half pint of Guinness – that were sacrificed.

As we shall see with subjective views of health, people may be reluctant to portray themselves as in need. Although this is probably so at all ages, it may increase with old age. Moreover, individuals may make comparisons concerning their standard of living, not only with those of their own age, but with their relatives, or their own childhood and youth in years gone by. Certainly, disguising poverty may have been less easy in the distant days of their youth as the old jingle suggests:

When you're living down poverty street
Everyone knows you're poor

Seen from this viewpoint, the poverty of the past may make present circumstances appear superior to someone aged 90 and over. It is these experiences and perceptions that create difficulties with the concept of relative deprivation (Townsend 1979), where new indicators are used in developing 'objective assessments'. These indicators are important in keeping alive the debate about poverty among the elderly though, as Townsend himself has recently shown, increasing material deprivation among the very old can be combined with self-perceptions showing that they feel better able to manage than younger people (Townsend 1989: Tables 3, 5). From our own evidence, the majority among our sample did not, and clearly did not want to, define themselves as poor, even though they might well have appreciated better living standards.

WHERE LIVING

Over half our sample had always lived in the immediate locality we found them in. Of the eight study areas three were predominantly

Table 2.4 Type of residence by sex: weighted sample

Type of residence	Women %	Men %
Private households	45.6	57.5
Communal establishments	54.4	42.5
Total	100	100
	(160)	(40)

rural, three predominantly urban and two mixed urban–rural. Urban backgrounds were reported by the majority of the sample members.

Moving from the general to the particular, very old people are less likely than younger old people still to be living in private households. Our total sample divided more or less evenly between the two main types of accommodation – 49 per cent living in private households and 51 per cent in communal establishments, though, as between women and men there is a marked difference (see Table 2.4).

Taking the actual sample, it is evident that the transfer from a private household to some form of communal living increases with age (see Appendix 2, Table A2.2). Three-quarters of the twelve centenarians had made the transition. Although it applies to both sexes, it is predominantly among the women that what appears to be a precipitator of residential accommodation – advancing years, with its probable corollary of increasing frailty – can be detected to the greatest extent. We now look more closely at the living arrangements of people over 90 years of age.

LIVING IN PRIVATE HOUSEHOLDS

The two broad categories of private households and communal establishments outlined previously mask important differences, as we shall see in later chapters, in the possibilities for care and companionship, in degrees of dependency and responsibility and in the extent to which elderly people are subject to risk. Here, we set the scene.

Who living with

To live alone at the age of 90 or more suggests a considerable degree of good health and independence. And this is no unusual happening. As

Table 2.5 Household composition of those in private households by sex: weighted sample

Who living with	Women %	Men %	Total %
Alone	42.7	33.3	40.4
With: children	38.7	25.0	35.4
siblings/other			
relatives/friends	9.3	16.7	11.1
spouse	–	20.8	5.0
In sheltered housing	9.3	4.2	8.1
Total	100	100	100
	(74)	(24)	(98)

can be seen in Table 2.5, the largest single group – two-fifths of those in private households – were, in fact, living alone. This compares with over half of those aged 85 and over in the general population (OPCS 1989: Table 12.2) and just over three-fifths of those aged 85 and over living in an inner-city London area (Bowling *et al.* 1988: 18).

Those living alone consisted mainly of women and men aged 90–94, and they constituted nearly half the former and well over a third of the latter. Among those aged 95 and over living alone was Mrs Chester, who lived independently under what many consider ideal conditions – in a 'granny flat' attached to her son's house.

A substantial minority of the sample members, as we would expect, were living with their children, more women, proportionately, than men, as is generally found (Victor, 1987: 219). The word 'children' conjures up a rather different image from the reality of sons and daughters in our study, themselves in most cases of pensionable age, a few in their seventies (their average age was 64), some with health problems of their own or with ailing spouses. In some cases, the parent maintained a real independence in daily living activities even though they lived with a daughter or son and daughter-in-law; in others they were totally dependent. The majority in this group could be described as semi-dependent, in the sense that they represented a whole range of conditions and circumstances, only some of which required the continuous help of others.

Eight per cent of our sample were living in sheltered housing accommodation. This category presents difficulties. At the time of the 1981 census, if 'at least half the people within a sheltered housing complex possessed facilities for cooking their own meals all were treated as members of private households, and, if less than half, they were treated as members of communal establishments' (OPCS 1983b). The Wagner Report (1988) included brief references to sheltered housing and 'very sheltered housing', thus placing it in the category of residential care. On the other hand, The Griffiths Report (1988), concerned with community-care policy also included the provision of sheltered housing among its options. In the present study, because of the small numbers, we decided to resolve the dilemma of hybrid residential/community status of sheltered housing by placing it under the private-household umbrella.

Everything today, we are told, must be done to discourage the 'dependency culture'. Housing elderly people in special units where they can, to all intents and purposes, maintain their independence, though with fewer responsibilities, satisfies official policy. At the same time, given the wherewithal to make choices, it can prove satisfactory for elderly people themselves. Approximately 5 per cent of the elderly population (Victor 1987: 140) do opt for the alternative of sheltered housing and, with an ever-increasing number of private developments for those who can afford it, the proportions will increase correspondingly.

In recent years, however, there has been a strong thread of criticism running through the relevant research and informed comment (see e.g. Attenburrow 1976; Butler et al. 1983; Middleton 1987; Pooley 1988). Even the Wagner Committee, despite their opinion that the strong demand for sheltered housing is surely here to stay, thought that it might 'reflect to some extent the inadequacy of support services to people in their own homes, rather than a real preference for a sheltered way of life' (Wagner 1988: 20).

Although the proportions of elderly people living alone have risen sharply during the course of this century (Victor 1987: 219), it is not a new phenomenon. Similarly, though the historical myth of the idealized extended family all living together has been exploded (see e.g. Laslett 1972 and, more recently, Gordon 1989: 303), living with children is not a new idea. What is new is the possible age to which many more people now live, with the consequence that these various living arrangements may endure for many years or need to be changed as increased frailty renders them unsuitable. What is also new in the context of living arrangements is the upsurge of home ownership.

Tenure

Before the First World War, when our study members were in their early youth, 'so little interest was taken in owner occupation that no contemporary figures exist about the numbers of owner-occupiers' (DOE 1977: para 1.90). They and their families, along with the vast majority of the population, would have been tenants of private landlords or, if working on the land, living in tied cottages. With the appearance of local authority housing in 1919, publicly-subsidized housing as a welfare service was born. In subsequent years private ownership became more and more a financially and socially desirable goal. Now, at 63 per cent of all tenures (CSO 1989a: Table 8.21) it dominates the housing scene.

Elderly people share in this preponderance but, generally, to a lesser degree, since, the older they are the more likely they are to have made decisions about their housing 'before the institution of government policies, most notably tax relief on mortgages, designed to encourage the large-scale growth of home ownership' (Victor, 1987: 130). The *very* old, however, as evidenced by our sample members, are more likely than not to be living in owned homes, including a few owned by relatives. This applied to 69 per cent of the sample in private households (we do not know of the housing tenure of the previous homes of those now in communal establishments).

If, however, home ownership is considered according to social class, the discrepancies between national levels and those of our sample lessen. Ninety per cent and 83 per cent, respectively, belonging to the Registrar-General classes I and II (with economically active household heads) are owner-occupiers (either outright or as mortgagees) compared with 68 per cent and 63 per cent respectively for classes III(i) and (ii) and 39 per cent and 29 per cent respectively for classes IV and V (CSO 1989a).

Seventeen per cent of those in the private-household sample were living in local council houses or flats at the time of the interview. This compares with 27 per cent of the population at large (ibid).

Housing type and amenities

The relative level of affluence of some of the sample members is again reflected in the type of housing and standards of the amenities they enjoyed. Thus, one-third of the domiciliary-based sample lived in semi-detached houses and just under a third in detached. One-fifth lived in terraced houses and the remainder in a flat, purpose-built or converted.

The great majority of homes had a garden, even if only a small one. This is of particular significance to individuals whose mobility is restricted, as was apparent in replies to a question put to our sample on things giving pleasure. Even 'houseboundness' might not preclude the possibility of a gentle excursion into the garden. But were it to do so, much enjoyment may be gained from its contemplation, as was so for Dr Carey, who got 'great pleasure' from his garden and knowing he did 'not have to work in it'.

Within doors, also, people ageing roughly parallel with the century will have seen enormous changes, and again we have to ask ourselves what these changes meant to them. Even for a younger generation being brought up just after the Second World War, 'the old tin bath', 'the pot under the bed' when it was too cold in the night to go outside to the WC, the 'bottom drawer' in lieu of a cot, visits to the public wash house, were all associated with nostalgic, happy memories of childhood (Holme 1985: 124). For someone very old, and possibly frail, household comforts must be a plus. Nevertheless if, like Mrs Sutton, you 'have been used to no inside toilet' all your life, you might well, with her, say 'it doesn't worry me'.

Mrs Benson and Mrs Baines both lived alone and were without any running hot water as well as no inside WC. The former wished to move and the interviewer thought her accommodation unsuitable, particularly as she had difficulty in walking. Mrs Baines, by contrast, wished only to remain in the home she had lived in most of her life. There were altogether four homes in the actual sample without permanent running hot water and five without a fixed bath or shower. The problem of incontinence must be greatly exacerbated by the lack of running hot water in the house, as was the case with Mrs Cross, aged 95, who wetted the bed at night. Small though the numbers are, the existence in the 1980s of any inadequately plumbed homes lived in by very old people must give cause for concern.

But whether judged by such standards or by those of our own interviewers, the amenities and the quality of the living arrangements were relatively good. As far as was possible to tell during summertime visits, the interviewers found very little to criticize about heating arrangements. Internally, three-quarters of the homes were, in their view, in good or very good condition.

It is not, of course, only the condition of the plumbing or the decorative order that determine the suitability or otherwise of a dwelling. Another factor which needs to be taken into account for very old people, many of whom have limited mobility, is convenience for moving about, and inconvenience in one form or another was the main reason given for the unsuitability of a home. In general terms, the interviewers assessed 51 per cent of the private households as 'very suitable' and a further 36 per cent as 'fairly suitable'; as many as 57 per cent were considered to be of high quality and as few as 5 per cent of poor quality.

Length of residence

We have already seen that many people in their 90s and beyond tend to stay put in their localities. The same is true of the length of time in their homes.

Well over half the total sample in private households had been in their present homes for more than fifteen years, nearly half of these for thirty-six years or more. Seven per cent of this group had not moved for over sixty years. It was evident from many of the replies that this stability was deeply valued. Not suprisingly, such a long period of residence was in notable contrast to that of people living in communal establishments.

LIVING IN COMMUNAL ESTABLISHMENTS

Length of residence

The vast majority of the individuals in residential accommodation of one kind or another had been there for only four years or less and most of these for under two years. This suggests that, in general, entry into residential care by members of the cohort is, for one reason or another, postponed for as long as possible. Thereafter, the rate of entry seems steadily to increase.

In spite of the relatively short duration of their sojourn in such places, it was evident that, just as with the private-household sample, once there, there was little desire among the majority for change. Miss Spencer, for instance, had made the transition four years previously after a spell in hospital following eighty-nine years of residence in her own home. She was now thoroughly settled, with a room of her own and within reasonable distance of her cousin.

In a consideration of very old people living in communal establishments, it is important to remember first, that there will be a sizeable group who are unable (or unwilling) to give their views, those, for instance, suffering from severe confusion or dementia. This applied to a quarter of the 'communal' sample compared with only a small fraction of those living at home. Secondly, our earlier word of caution about elderly people not wishing to complain must apply with particular force to those in residential care. With our sample, every effort was made to maintain privacy during the interview and its confidential nature was naturally stressed. Furthermore, we were able, to some extent, to rely on the impartial assessments of the interviewers, whose access to the homes or hospitals often took them into bedrooms or wards as well as public rooms. Nevertheless, there must be some reservations.

Type of communal establishment

Broadly, there are three main types of communal establishment to which elderly people may go for long-term care – residential homes, nursing homes and hospitals – but within these three categories there are further divisions. Is there nursing care, for instance, in the residential home? Does the hospital provide psychiatric or simply 'geriatric' care? Is the establishment run by a local authority, the National Health Service or is it owned privately for profit or by a voluntary agency? Following Day and Klein (1987: 384) and Harman and Harman (1989), our definition of private provision includes voluntary homes, of which there were only a few in the sample. The distinction between the private and statutory sectors these days is in some respects a narrow one, since the 'private' resident or patient may be subsidized by the DHSS. In total, supplementary-benefit/income-support subsidies for accommodation had escalated to nearly £900 million per year by 1988 (ibid.: 157).

In our study, we found that more sample members were in private (and voluntary) residential homes and nursing homes than in homes run by the local authority (see Table 2.6). Although the proportions of the former group are somewhat higher than might be expected (see e.g. Victor 1987: 292–295) they may well be accounted for by the rapidity of the increase in the private sector.

A further analysis of the local authority homes showed the majority to be without nursing care.

Clearly, the three main types of establishment – residential home, nursing home and hospital – carry with them different types of organization and a different spread of amenities; furthermore, between the individual establishments we should expect to find differences. Leaving aside hospital provision for the moment, we also looked to see

Table 2.6 Residence in different types of communal establishment by sex: weighted sample

Type of communal establishments	Women %	Men %	Total %
Local authority residential, with and without nursing care	27.9	43.8	30.4
Private residential	27.9	25.0	27.5
Private nursing home	24.4	18.8	23.5
Hospital:			
geriatric/psychiatric	12.8	12.4	12.7
cottage/GP/private	7.0	–	5.8
Total	100	100	100[1]
	(86)	(16)	(102)

[1]See note 2.

if there were differences apparent between privately run and publicly run homes.

Over half the sample had a room to themselves and this was no less the case in council-run homes than private ones; similarly with the sharing of a bathroom or WC. There was, however, one difference. Only just over two-thirds of the local council residents compared with over four-fifths of those in private residential or nursing homes had furniture or fittings of their own.

For an assessment generally of quality and suitability of the communal establishments of our sample, we have relied in the main on the common-sense opinions of the interviewers, supplemented, of course, by the views of the elderly people themselves, which we take up in later chapters. Of the total number – eighty-six – of communal establishments of all kinds (see note 3) fourteen were said by the interviewers to be of poor quality; twelve had a 'poor atmosphere', with strict rules, little autonomy or choice and nothing extra done for the patients or residents. No one type of establishment – local authority, voluntary or private – predominated in this assessment. There was also a handful of places which received neutral comment – they were 'fairly suitable', had an 'efficient' but evidently not a particularly warm or caring regime.

Against such adverse or neutral comments by the interviewers must be set some mixed and many glowing accounts of establishments where

41

the regimes were 'flexible and free', 'easy going', had a 'pleasant' or 'very pleasant atmosphere'.

The external and internal conditions of the majority of the communal establishments were highly regarded by the interviewers. There was, however, criticism of a greater proportion of them, irrespective of their private or public status, than of private households. This focused on the quality of the living arrangements, their organization and relations between staff and resident or patient. We return to this topic in Chapter 8.

As with other spheres of the study, it does not necessarily follow that a home – private or communal – assessed by an outside observer as 'suitable' or 'unsuitable' is seen in the same light by the person most intimately concerned. Clearly, as we shall see in later chapters, satisfactions or dissatisfactions about living arrangements and standards of care are vital components of the quality of everyday life, and may influence, or be influenced by, the ability to choose where and how to live.

SUMMARY

In so far as the sample of nonagenarians and centenarians is representative of people of those ages in England, we can say with confidence that they differ markedly from younger people in many important ways. Women predominate in significantly greater numbers; widowhood even more so. Social-class position tends more to the middle and higher ranks than generally in the population, and there is relatively less poverty. Proportionately many more have crossed the great divide between home and Home, almost certainly for good. The interviewers assessed the standard of both kinds of accommodation, with some exceptions, as reasonably good, a view, as we shall see later, shared by the majority of the elderly people themselves. The exceptions on both counts, however, must not be overlooked.

There is, then, heterogeneity among people aged 90 and over, even in their basic social and residential circumstances. Nevertheless, their many similarities of characteristics and circumstances make them a coherent group. Perhaps what makes them unique as a group is their shared experience of the First World War and the extent of social and economic change which has occurred during the course of their long lives. This we take up again in the next chapter.

3

LONGEVITY AND POSSIBLE INFLUENCES

It is a popular belief, but a fallacy, that we can learn about what contributes to extreme old age by studying very old survivors. This certainly needs to be done, but it is also necessary to know about the characteristics of other members of their birth cohort, in early childhood, adulthood and early old age. In this chapter we can say quite a lot about those surviving to the age of 90 and beyond, but in order to compare them with their contemporaries, who did not survive through earlier stages of the life course, we would need to undertake a job of reconstruction from data sources, many of which are inadequate.

We have attempted some reconstruction in this chapter, but, inevitably, our data are often sparse. Conclusions, therefore, are sparing and at times somewhat speculative. Above all, we need to make the point again that social experiences (including public events and private life styles) were not the same as those of previous cohorts; and no subsequent one will have had a comparable set of experiences either. In short, though it is a popular pastime, there has to be great caution in making any statement about what does or does not promote extreme longevity.

We begin by discussing in more detail the 'life-course' concept, introduced earlier, and illustrate further, using the words of our study members, some of the dramatic changes in circumstances and experiences which have occurred in the twentieth century. In so doing we provide an outline of the historical *context* of survival into very old age.

We then consider three types of our survey *evidence* about survival. First, we examine the possible influences of biological factors. Secondly, these are contrasted with social influences on survival (including those of life style and behaviour), though it will be clear that the separation of biological and social factors is, in some respects, arbitrary. Thirdly, we consider what the sample members themselves

43

think about surviving into very old age; what factors they think have been important and whether they are pleased that it has occurred.

THE LIFE COURSE: HISTORICAL AND BIOGRAPHICAL

The 'life tree' that follows lists those events likely to have been the most important in the public sphere and in the private lives of the people in our survey. Of course, this life tree is an abstraction of a limited range of events. The reader might, however, find it useful as a backdrop to what follows.

The formative years of the people in our sample were clearly dominated by the transition from the Victorian age to that of Edward VII and the enormous impact of the First World War. Since that time, just as the economic and social situation seemed to be easing towards the end of the 1930s, the world was engulfing them, and now their children, in another global conflict. By the time of full employment and post-war prosperity the people in our study were already moving into the last stages of their working lives.

It was not, however, only major events that made their mark. There were, as we saw in Chapter 2, the continuing, accelerating social and technological changes – large and small, and impelled by an ever-growing population – that affected the way of life of people of all ages. A steady decline in the impact of disease on children and young adults was especially important.

In this connection, changes in public health provision were remembered by members of our sample. Mrs Warner was one.

> My daughter says the water's not good around here – it goes slimy in the glass if you leave it. I said to her, 'Well, dear, where I lived we used to go down to a little old spring and there was all green stuff on it and we used to have to scrape that all off before we got our bucket of water. There was no pump.'

Other changes in circumstances and behaviour were highlighted. Mrs King described her husband in the early days of their marriage. 'He was a tough little character and had a strict mother. After we were married he was very much the master. He wouldn't allow me to do anything if he said I hadn't to do it.' Mrs Pollard, aged 100, remembered that 'those days you didn't live with a man as soon as you left school'.

In answer to a question asking them to compare past and present, those preferring the past talked of the present-day increase in crime, of

Life tree

	Historical/public events	Personal events
1881–1913	End of Victorian era Boer War Edwardian era Introduction of social insurance	Birth Childhood

1914–1918	First World War	War service, death of
		  brothers
		  husbands, loved ones
		Marriage

1919–1929	Influenza epidemic Economic crisis General strike	Family building
1930–1938	The Depression International tensions	Approaching high point of employment/career
1939–1945	Second World War	Own and children's war service
1950–1969	'Full employment' Rapid social change Rising living standards Developing technology	Children leave, marry Grandchildren Retirement

1970–
present
	Rising unemployment
	Oil crisis
	End of political
	  consensus
	Thatcher years
		Death of spouse, siblings,
		  friends
		Entering very old age

rudeness and violence amongst the young, 'people were more contented then'. Dr Carey thought 'the friendly neighbour was very rare [nowadays]'.

In my practice before the war I had a list of about twenty women I could call on who were quite willing to go and spend the night with people who were ill and keep an eye on them, and most of them did it for nothing.

Echoing a finding from the study of *Family and Kinship in East London* (Young and Willmott 1957), he blamed this change on 'the complete alteration of the housing. You see, the terraced house is far the best type of house for people with low incomes and these people, with exceptions, were all friendly and were able to help each other.'

Mr Crawford thought that present-day life was more of a rat race and he believed he would 'enjoy it less'. 'The young', he thought, 'are not so good because of circumstances. The average teenager has lost all respect for things we called respectable.'

Mrs Forbes expressed the views of a small, well-to-do group.

It was better fifty years ago because we would have had our own servants to look after us; an old nanny or someone. If it had been years ago I shouldn't be in this place. Now you can't get anybody. Not even a housekeeper.

These reminiscences not only describe the past but also reconstruct it, sometimes contrasting it with certain features of present-day life which they found unacceptable. In this way a sense of common values held by survivors of a generation can be reinforced (Williams 1986). Such reminiscences, as we saw in Chapter 2, are of course open to the charge that they represent a myth of a golden age which may often play down the realities of hardship and social tensions (Roberts 1973). But this does not diminish their importance. Such accounts, by stressing periods in the past which entailed activity and involvement, may reflect a loss of role and responsibility experienced in very old age.

The dominant theme among those preferring the present centred on the welfare state. 'The National Health Service means better medical care, wonderful nurses, no worries generally.' 'Nowadays you don't have to depend on relatives.' Shades of the workhouse were evoked. 'They worked until the day they died, in those days.'

Mr Craddock's views were along these lines:

People nowadays are provided for when they are old. I remember the time when the first five shillings was given to the pensioner; up to that time they got nothing. They used to rely on their daughters or sons or somebody. I remember my grand-mother, she was pleased as punch when she got her five shillings pension.

Mr Unwin praised modern conveniences – 'electric light and the telephone and the rest of it certainly ease life'.

In sum these comments provide a stock of 'generational knowledge' which links key features of the social structure to those of personal experience. It is within this 'life-course' context that specific influences on survival should be considered.

BIOLOGICAL INFLUENCES

Childhood health

A degree of historical imagination is needed to grasp the changes in childhood health since the end of the last century. Today, public concern is with (thankfully rare) serious conditions, many of which are genetic in origin. In developed nations, the infections are largely noticeable by their absence or by their reduction in virulence, though certainly vigilance is required to ensure that they do not undergo a resurgence (Dubos 1960).

In the last part of the nineteenth century and first part of the twentieth, epidemics of scarlet fever, diphtheria and measles were common among children. Indeed, in examining a 'log book' for a South London primary school in the 1930s, one of the present authors has recently observed large and regular absences from school, sometimes as much as 30 per cent, due to measles. Whooping cough has continued to dog our heels even into modern times, and outbreaks of poliomyelitis in the 1950s shocked the British public out of their complacency about the infections. And, of course, AIDS has now shocked a new generation into an understanding of what fatal infectious disease can mean.

Nonetheless, these phenomena bear little comparison with earlier periods, including the years in which the people in our study were growing up. As Winter (1985: 14) puts it 'there were conditions of poverty and ill health that today we associate with countries of the third world'. Rowntree (1901) had shown that between 3 and 4 million people in Britain – 10 per cent of the population – could not buy enough food to sustain normal activities, and inspectorates pointed out that chronic malnutrition was widespread among low wage labourers (Winter 1985: 17–18).

It was fortunate indeed for a working-class child to survive both the period immediately after birth and then the early years of life. For those that did survive, there is increasing evidence that poor social conditions and poor health in childhood might have a marked effect on

47

adult health and indeed on survival (see e.g. Marmot *et al.* 1987: 128). From this viewpoint, the individuals in our study might be more appropriately seen as exceptional survivors of a birth cohort of children, many of whom did not survive into adult life, or, if they did, succombed in early or late working life.

The evidence, however, from the picture of childhood health reported by our interviewees, suggests that they had been able for the most part to escape the ravages wrought by childhood infections or deficiency diseases. When asked to rate their childhood health status, nearly 75 per cent replied that it was 'very good' with a further 17 per cent rating it as 'fairly good' and less than one in ten as 'poor'. This positive view is further borne out by the very low proportions of illnesses the sample remembered occurring in childhood. Furthermore, when asked about their adult life, their health seems to have continued to be good, with only 4 per cent saying that it was 'poor'.

It appears, then, that in contrast to many of their generation our long-lived survivors may have started out with the head start of a healthy childhood. While the conditions of urban working-class life had a devastating effect on the mass of the population, those in relative affluence were much more likely to be able to withstand or avoid the worst of the potential hazards from infectious and other diseases. Winter (1985: 9), for example, cites an infant mortality rate (the number of deaths in the first year of life for every 1,000 births) in Hampstead in 1910 as 60, whereas in areas such as Birmingham, Blackburn, Burnley, Dudley (one of the areas of our present study) Preston, and Wakefield the figure was 200 per 1,000 births.

Clearly, to have weathered these early storms was already a matter of 'survivorship' in itself, particularly if coming from working-class or poor backgrounds. Moreover, the interaction of biological and 'confounding' social factors is once again in evidence. If, as appears from their childhood-health history, our sample members are to some extent distinguished from others born around the same time, were there also distinctions in the longevity of their parents?

Long-lived forebears

There is a saying that in order to live a long life it is preferable to choose long-lived parents. Sometimes it is held that the effect works better if the survival of grandparents rather than parents is taken as the keystone, as if longevity worked by generational skips. People thus search their family trees, if not the palms of their hands for long life.

Table 3.1 Age at death of fathers by sex: weighted sample

Father's age at death	Women %	Men %
39 and under	3.2	3.0
40–69	34.9	27.3
70–79	23.8	30.3
80–89	31.8	27.3
90+	6.3	12.1
Total subjects	100	100
	(126)	(33)

Not only that, but stories of people in other parts of the world also occur frequently in the mass media, even though there is little supporting evidence in the shape, for instance, of birth certificates.

How do these popular ideas stand up in relation to our survey findings, at least as far as forebears are concerned? Information on grandparents from our survey is unfortunately limited, but of 114 members of the actual sample three-quarters said they had one or more 'long-lived grandparent'.

Turning to parents, as can be seen in Table 3.1 a substantial proportion of fathers did indeed live into old age. Some 70 per cent of the men's fathers, and 62 per cent of the women's, lived to be over 70 years of age; 39 per cent and 38 per cent, respectively, lived to the age of 80 or beyond.

A picture, similar in essence though differing in particulars, emerges from the reported ages at death of the mothers of our sample members, as shown in Table 3.2. Here 78 per cent of mothers of the men, and 80 per cent of those of the women, had lived to at least the age of 70 with no less than 40 per cent and 47 per cent respectively, living to the age of 80 and beyond. The mothers' average age at death of the six female centenarians replying to the question was 83.

It appears, then, that a substantial proportion of our sample did have long-lived parents. Inevitably, however, there is a need for caution in interpreting such figures. First, not all members of the sample were able to recall the ages at death of their parents. It is possible that those unable to reply or remember would have had parents who died at a younger age.

Secondly, it is not entirely surprising that most of the sample's parents appear to have lived to a reasonable old age, given the fact that

Table 3.2 Age at death of mothers by sex: weighted sample

Mother's age at death	Women %	Men %
39 and under	6.8	6.3
40–69	13.6	15.6
70–79	32.6	40.6
80–89	35.6	25.0
90+	11.4	12.5
	100	100
Total subjects	(131)	(32)

life expectancy of anyone surviving childhood has always been much higher than life expectancy at birth. The parents of our study group, by definition, had of course done just this. As a guide it is worth noting that the additional expected years of life for people aged 30 in the year 1900 was 35 years, (i.e. a life expectancy of 65 years) considerably more than is sometimes popularly supposed.

Given the fact that 65 is an *average* figure we would expect some individuals to survive into very old age, though steeply rising death rates above that age (especially for the period in question) would be likely to reduce the numbers considerably over the age of 80. Certainly, the proportion of the population alive over the age of 80 at any one time has been very small indeed throughout this century; for example, the figure in 1951 was less than 2 per cent (CSO 1955). Whilst such figures cannot be used in any direct way to shed light on our parents' survival pattern (as we do not know how many of the parents were alive at any one point in time), we feel that it is reasonable to conclude from the distribution of the parents' ages of death that proportionately more survived into very old age than the population in general.

As we can see, the picture is not a simple one, largely because we are not dealing with the survival of a random sample of the original cohort. We discuss later the effects of social class on survival, and it is clear from this that class may be a confounding factor in mapping the influence of inherited characteristics.

Long-lived brothers and sisters

The ability to remember the age of their parents at their death was less in evidence in the case of brothers and sisters. This is regrettable from the viewpoint of the present discussion, since siblings in many respects are a more reliable source of comparison than parents, as they share the same parents (Clarke 1987). Many of the people in our study had lost touch with siblings during their lives; others were simply unable to remember exactly what had happened to all of them. This is not perhaps surprising given a very long life and the fact that, of the 176 members of the actual sample replying, as many as 77 per cent had at least three siblings and not far short of one-third had seven or more.

One of the most important confounding historical factors at work in any attempt to look at the siblings' longevity is the impact of war. The effects of the First World War on the demographic structure of Britain is still controversial (see, in particular, Winter 1985). It is now estimated that some three-quarters of a million British men died in that war, including a 'lost generation' of upper-class, as well as a massive loss of working-class, men. Nearly one-third of the identified brothers in our sample were reported to have died as a direct result of war.

Allowing for the problems – biographical and historical – of assessing the longevity of siblings based on self-reports, we were still presented with a relatively clear picture of long-lived siblings, especially sisters. The fact that sisters' ages at death appear consistently higher than those of brothers (see Appendix 2, Tables A2.3 and A2.4) ties in with the known superior survival pattern of women compared with men in recent times. Altogether, 39 per cent of the sample women's sisters were reported to have lived to the age of 80 and beyond, and 38 per cent of the sample men's sisters. The figures for brothers were 28 per cent and 16 per cent, respectively.

The question of sex

As has been clear from the outset, the influence of sex has been considerable. By the age of 90, eight out of ten survivors are women. Table 3.3 shows that sex differences in survival grow more apparent throughout the later part of the life course, as the result of a marked increase in deaths amongst men between the ages of 50 and 79 (for a fuller discussion see Baylis et al. 1986; Clarke 1986).

This increase in male deaths in later middle age and early old age is due in large measure to the much higher rates of heart disease in late-middle-aged men and is especially evident amongst manual workers, contrary to the persistent belief that heart disease is a disease of affluence (Marmot et al. 1978). Lung cancer and respiratory disease also take their toll in later life amongst men. Whilst in western society

Table 3.3 Death rates per 1000 population by age and sex 1986

Age groups	Male	Female
25–34	0.9	0.5
35–44	1.7	1.1
45–54	5.5	3.3
55–64	17.0	9.5
65–74	43.6	24.0
75–84	102.0	63.2
85+	217.1	172.4

Source: CSO 1989[b], Table 2.22.

death rates for males are higher than for females, morbidity rates, especially those for mental illness, appear to be higher for women. The influence of biological factors in mortality and morbidity in adult life is thus compounded by social and occupational factors (Powles 1978) and the differences between men's and women's social roles (Nathanson 1975).

Of possible interest here in extending our appreciation of the interaction of biological and social factors, is the question of marriage.

SOCIAL FACTORS

Marriage

There is some evidence in the literature to suggest that whilst marriage seems to act as a protector in terms of physical and mental health for both men and women, it does so more for men than for women (Gove 1973). Men are more likely to react poorly to bereavement, for example, in both their mental health and their survival (Bowling *et al.* 1988). Furthermore, as we have seen, they are more likely than women to remarry.

For women, marriage itself carries many hazards, both in terms of 'gender roles' and those which they may be exposed to throughout their lives, most notably, of course, child bearing. The difficulty here, is to identify the specific influences and the particular points in the life course at which they may have occurred.

It seems clear from the evidence presented so far in this chapter that whatever the mix of biological and social factors at work in promoting longevity, they are expressed in family structures. Running concurrently with this picture is the influence of social class.

Social class

There is an accumulation of evidence that the place occupied in the social structure has a strong association with health and particularly 'premature' mortality (MacIntyre 1986; Townsend et al. 1988). It is equally true, however, that the interpretation of such observed inequalities, especially when they are used as evidence of trends over a period of time, is hotly disputed. This is because social class, in one sense, is a 'construct' as well as a part of experience; definitions of it may, and do, change and it becomes particularly difficult to compare one period with another because of social mobility (Illsley 1980). The occupations which denote membership of one social class at a point in time (as classified for official purposes) may be replaced by other occupations at a later point due to technological and other changes.

When we try to assess the impact of social class on the chances of surviving into very old age we face even more difficult problems. We might expect, for example, that the influence of social class on survival would gradually diminish with age. Those from higher social classes are more likely initially to survive, and those from lower social classes who do so might represent a highly selected group of particularly fit individuals. Yet recent evidence has shown that inequalities persist in mortality between social classes well beyond the statutory retirement age (Fox et al. 1985), suggesting that social class not only affects the selection process into very old age, but the experience of life once there.

Two factors in particular interfere with attempts to assess the impact of social class on longevity. First is the enormous change in the industrial and occupational structure, the relative fall in the proportion of the population in manual occupations and the rise in non-manual occupations, especially for women, in the labour market. These changes make any comparison between the very old and other age groups particularly difficult. Very old people have experienced both changes in their own career patterns across the 'life course' and the historical changes in occupational structure.

Second is the social position of women. Their changing pattern of employment, including their highly variable involvement in paid work, creates particular difficulties for sociological analysis. For our study group, this applies with even more force when we consider the fact that 80 per cent of the weighted sample are women and that their possible working lives, spanning anything from two to fifty years, finished, with one or two exceptions, at least thirty years ago.

Many complexities surrounded the working lives of the women of our sample. Moreover, a substantial minority had never worked. For these reasons and others, including the need to make comparisons with national data, we decided, as noted in Chapter 2, to employ the traditional classification.

The main question at this point is how far do those aged 90 and over differ in their social class from the general population, and, therefore, how far can we say that longevity is associated with social position? Two broad comparisons are perhaps the most useful, namely how far the people in our sample differed from the population in the earlier part of this century, and how far they differ from the population today.

In 1911, when our sample was entering the labour market, the census shows that 80 per cent of the population were in manual occupations. This compares with 50 per cent in our sample (see Chapter 2, Table 2.2). In 1981 the situation for the population as a whole had changed considerably, with a smaller proportion in manual occupations, and a larger in classes I and II. For example, only 14 per cent of the population were classified as being in classes I and II in 1911 compared with 25 per cent in 1981 and no less than 35 per cent in our own sample. (Census data are taken from Abercrombie *et al* 1988: 118–121.)

These comparisons underpin our earlier contention that the majority of our sample of people surviving to the age of 90 and beyond are from the middle ranks, with a significantly larger minority in social class I than is to be found in the general population. Moreover, the proportions of men in our study in the unskilled manual category is extremely small, as we would expect from the marked increase in mortality for working-class men in late middle age and early old age. As we have noted, however, losses in the First World War fell disproportionately on upper-class men (particularly those of subaltern rank) and this must have influenced the survival pattern of the birth cohort from which our men are drawn. For women the position is apparently more mixed, although, at the individual level it was clear from the interviewing that we were sometimes dealing with individuals of considerable means.

We think that the two processes we have discussed have been instrumental in creating this picture. On the one hand, it seems clear that a number (perhaps over one-half) of those living into very old age were born into relatively comfortable circumstances. They were unlikely from this viewpoint to have been exposed to the impact of poverty and the high risk from infectious disease in their early years. On the other hand, it is also clear that there has been a degree of social mobility over the life course which partly explains the current social position of those in our sample.

This last point is illustrated by comparing the evidence we have on father's occupation for the sample, with the sample's own social class (see Appendix 2, Table A2.5). Though the differences between the two groups are relatively small they are in line with the changes that have occurred in the twentieth century – especially an expansion of social class I and a reduction in social class IV. Additionally, it is clear that the fathers were more middle class than the population in general.

Life style

In any discussion of the impact of social position on survival, analysts are always open to the criticism that the argument is a deterministic one. In some respects this is inevitable. Some aspects of social position *do* determine life chances including survival. Nothing we have seen from our present study persuades us otherwise. Even so, we recognize that there has been a growing interest in personal behaviours which increase the risk of life-shortening diseases (particularly cardio-vascular diseases and cancer), even amongst those in medical and social research committed to an environmentalist perspective. Whilst it may be true that the emphasis on individual 'health promotion' is an elaborate attempt to 'blame the victim' (Crawford 1977; Townsend *et al.* 1988), the role of health-related behaviours cannot be dismissed in summary fashion.

Here again, however, the relevance of current trends to the study findings must be approached with care. As Brody (1985) has argued, evidence for the beneficial impact of health-promoting regimes on the health and quality of life of the elderly is thin indeed. We can imagine that this is likely to undergo considerable change in the next ten years, as cohorts enter the ranks of the elderly with different values, more consistent perhaps with the growth of the consumer health-conscious culture. Whether this is the case or not, we are bound to be sceptical of the effects of some current 'health promotion' on the very old, brought up under very different historical and cultural circumstances. Certain health-promoting or hazardous behaviours, however, may well have influenced survivors, as we see in the first of these that we now consider – smoking.

Smoking

As soon as we begin to look at an issue such as smoking, we are made aware of how far behaviours, which are largely seen as a matter of

Table 3.4 Smoking history by sex: weighted sample

	Women %	Men %
Never have	72.4	36.8
Did, but not now	27.6	60.5
Yes, now	0.0	2.6
	100	100[1]
Total subjects	(152)	(38)

[1]See note 2.

individual choice, are, in reality, also strongly socially patterned. This is especially the case when viewed historically. The smoking history of those in the present study is summarized in Table 3.4.

Table 3.4 shows that 37 per cent of men and no less than 72 per cent of women (including all the seven female centenarians) reported that they had never smoked. Of the five male centenarians, three smoked a pipe at the time of interviewing and Mr Chandler five mannikin cigars a day. Cigarettes had not figured to any great extent in their smoking history. In the population at large, however, during the first quarter of the present century, smoking among men was almost universal. Survey data from 1956 show that of men aged 50 years and over, as few as 7 per cent had never smoked (Wald *et al.* 1988).

Cigarette smoking had become very popular, particularly amongst middle-class and upper-class men; manufactured cigarettes were too expensive in the early years of their availability for the working-class pocket. At the same time, it was still extremely rare for women to smoke. This soon changed, on both counts.

First, the history of smoking amongst men has reversed the earlier social-class pattern of manufactured cigarette smoking. In 1984 only 17 per cent of men from professional backgrounds smoked cigarettes, compared with 49 per cent of unskilled manual workers (CSO 1988). Secondly, by 1948, 40 per cent of women were smoking, including 23 per cent of those over the age of 60 years. By 1984, 15 per cent of women from professional backgrounds and 36 per cent of women from unskilled manual backgrounds were smoking (ibid).

It is clear from the figures, therefore, that the people in our study, especially the women, were exceptionally abstinent; not one woman reported being a smoker at the time of interview, and very few had smoked more than one or two a day. The exception was one woman in

Table 3.5 Drinking history by sex: weighted sample

	Women %	Men %
Never have	25.0	23.7
Did, but not now	24.4	21.0
Yes, now	50.6	55.3
	100	100
Total subjects	(156)	(38)

the age group 90–94 who had smoked forty cigarettes a day throughout her adult life. Of the men who had smoked, the great majority spoke of fewer than fifteen cigarettes a day.

Alcohol

The role of alcohol in promoting or retarding longevity is more difficult to assess than that of tobacco. There are few commentators outside the tobacco industry who would seriously question the effects of smoking on survival. Our data give strong support to this view. This is not the case, however, with alcohol. Heavy drinking and alcohol dependence, from both a common sense and scientific viewpoint, clearly damage health and contribute to premature mortality (notably from liver disease). It cannot be said, however, that the low or total abstention from alcohol, unlike non-smoking, has the opposite effect. To be teetotal might confer moral status, but the recurrent debate in the epidemiological literature in some quarters concerning the possible *protective* role of low-level alcohol consumption has hitherto lent weight to a 'moderation' perspective.

As can be seen from Table 3.5, whilst approximately one-quarter of the sample members reported that they had been teetotal throughout their lives (including five of the seven female and two of the five male centenarians), the greater proportion of those who had drunk alcohol still did so – marginally more among the men (55 per cent) than the women.

Again, one has to bear in mind the historical situation regarding such behaviours. Smoking was rare among women; the consumption of alcohol less so. Certainly in the years before, and especially during, the First World War, alcoholic drink was widely available. In 1914, pubs were open from 5 a.m. to 12.30 a.m. in London and 6 a.m. to 10 p.m.

Table 3.6 Frequency of current drinking habits by sex: weighted sample

	Women %	Men %
Abstainer	48.7	44.7
Occasional	12.5	10.5
Infrequent light	10.5	10.5
Frequent light	28.3	29.0
Moderate	0.0	2.6
Heavier	0.0	2.6
Total	100	100[1]
	(152)	(38)

[1]See note 2.

elsewhere. 'Drinks for our brave boys' was the common cry of the period (Ferguson 1975). After the First World War the population became more temperate overall, but heavy beer drinking, especially in male working-class life, was widespread.

Just as the sample has a strongly non-smoking character to it, so, as Table 3.6 shows, low and moderate levels of consumption are the dominant feature observed with alcohol.

The differences between men and women are also in the expected direction, with proportionately more women reporting 'occasional' consumption than men, and no women reporting moderate or heavy drinking. Mrs Sharp, for instance, aged 102, still had an occasional 'small glass of wine' and Mrs Vernon, aged 100, the same once or twice a week. These current drinking patterns are worth comparing with those of the population as a whole (see Appendix 2, Table A2.6).

Clear gender differences in the national data are even more evident than in our survey, and this becomes more marked when age is taken into account. Figures for 1980 show that more people were abstainers over the age of 65; 9 per cent and 24 per cent respectively (Wilson 1980). Moreover, Wilson's survey found very few women drinking either moderately or heavily over the age of 65 years.

Our own somewhat limited evidence shows that low levels of alcohol consumption may not be incompatible with survival into old age. But establishing the full smoking and drinking history of the sample would have taken a study in itself, as would the question of dietary behaviour to which we now briefly turn.

Diet and other forms of self-care

The link between diet and health appears to be an obvious one, particularly as we know that seriously inadequate intakes of food lead directly to health crises. Malnutrition and starvation still haunt many of the world's populations. In western nations there has been a rise in all manner of folk and scientific information about the effects of dietary habits on well-being and survival.

At the same time it is again obvious that the confounding effects of historical change are very much to be seen in any assessment of diet. Biographical and social structural influences are closely intertwined. Not only do individuals alter their diets over their lives, but their personal preferences, the availability of foods, their costs and their perceived benefits have constantly changed throughout this century. Certainly, the indicators of infant and maternal mortality for these periods, and the state of health of men recruited to the Armed Forces at the time (10 per cent of men were regarded as completely unfit for service and over 40 per cent unfit for combat (Winter 1985: 55)), suggest that nutritional standards were often inadequate.

The rather limited picture of diet we were able to gather from the members of our sample must be set, therefore, against a backcloth of considerable complexity. Certainly their replies to various questions on their eating habits, past and present, showed little recognition of current dietary advice. Eighty-one per cent, for example, said that they ate meat daily; 69 per cent ate butter rather than margarine; only just over half had fresh fruit every day (see Appendix 2, Table A2.7 for a summary of the sample's intake of various foodstuffs).

Some expressed forceful views on the subject of diet and current trends. Dr Carey, for instance, an ex GP, first paid tribute to the value of penicillin, alcohol – the 'finest tonic' – and opium – 'one of the two best drugs'. He then went on to extol the virtues of moderation, with a side swipe at food fashions.

> The same people who are dead against alcohol are loading our central nervous system with drugs by the hundreds and they are doing much more damage than alcohol ever did. It is quite ridiculous just because a few people abuse alcohol – you might just as well stop people eating bread. A few people abuse bread and get very fat. All this diet business. If only they'd turn round and tell people just to say 'No thank you' and eat less of everything, instead of all this nonsense of too much butter, etc. Of course you can have too much of everything. The whole point is moderation.

Having been brought up in times characterized by hardship, scarcity and rationing, whether for themselves or others, a lack of interest in dieting is hardly surprising. We might also contend that if people have survived to such a great age, there cannot be much seriously wrong with their diet. It is equally true that the social background of the people in our study means that the stark effects of a poor diet through poverty would not have been a central experience though, judging from some accounts, there were exceptions. It is also worth remembering, in this connection, that meat and dairy products were highly valued in official as well as popular circles during the larger part of this century.

Half the total sample described their appetite today as 'good' or 'very good' and a further 27 per cent as 'fairly good'. As would be expected, however, the majority no longer ate as much as they used to; a good appetite does not for this age group demand large quantities of food. This, in itself, meets one of the tenets of the 'sensible' diet – moderation.

All this is not to say that positive measures for protecting and improving health cannot, and indeed should not, apply as much in extreme old age as in younger ages, despite the rather negative position on the possible benefits taken up by some researchers (e.g. Brody 1985). Others (see e.g. Gray 1988) are more positive and would decidedly approve of 97-year-old Mr Potter's measures to keep fit. 'I do exercises every morning and night [demonstrated to the interviewer]. I got 'em off the TV.'

Whether such activities improve or maintain physical functioning may be arguable. We incline to the view, however, that the possible psychological benefits at least may have favourable repercussions on the quality of life. Moreover, it must also be said that in answer to another question, as we shall now see, the elderly members of our sample showed themselves to be not indifferent to the merits of self-care.

PERSONAL VIEWS OF LONGEVITY

Any discussion of the possible influence of biological, social and behavioural factors on longevity must take into account the views of individuals themselves. Subjective views may be of particular importance in considering the choices individuals have made through their lifetimes within a broad social and cultural context.

As can be seen from Table 3.7, the people in our study gave

Table 3.7 Stated reasons for longevity: weighted sample

To do with	%
Way of life:	
moderation generally and in smoking and drinking only, clean living and/or good food, etc.	30.9
outdoor life, exercise, hard work, etc., only or with moderation and care	13.8
Temperament:	
combined with other influences	22.0
only	17.1
Heredity, singly or combined with other influences	8.1
Other reasons including 'a strong heart', 'just luck'	8.1
Total	100
	(124)

considerable weight to factors that have arisen so far in our discussion, such as their way of life, and played down others. Thus they seemed to set relatively little store by the ages at death of parents and siblings that they had so notably remembered, though 'good stock' or its equivalent was mentioned by a few.

There were many specific as well as general references to their way of life; total abstinence figured prominently here. Mr Charles said that it depended on

> how you live and whether you look after yourself or whether you just let yourself go any old how. If you have got the will-power you can do a lot. You can see them now, the place [his residential home] is full of cripples and they're nearly all drinkers.

Although their way of life, or aspects of it, was given relatively often as a reason for their longevity, the message coming through their statements was less one of an explicit claim to 'moral worth' than of a fact of life. This is not to say that implicit moralizing attitudes of the kind were absent from some of the replies. The phrase 'clean living', after all, carries such connotations, as does 'hard work' or 'a Christian outlook'. They, or their equivalents, were used by about one-fifth of the sample. Similarly, when positive aspects of 'temperament' were invoked, as was the case by over one-fifth of the sample, it was more as an example of good fortune than moral virtue, though this last could sometimes be detected.

Mrs Horden gave priority to her 'contentment', plus 'a cooked meal every day'. She added that 'a lot of it is to do with will-power. Some days I don't really feel too good, but you haven't got to give way, have you?' Mrs Forbes gave as her reasons that she liked 'her fellowmen' and Mrs Hopkins that she had 'always done what [she] wanted to do'.

Dr Carey thought his long life had to do with 'chewing your food and real exercise when young. If you had to get somewhere you walked or cycled.' Three of the twelve centenarians attributed their great age to 'hard work'. Mr Dale talked of his heart. 'If that's no good you're no good and that's what's kept me alive, my heart. An artful chap! There's one thing about me, I'm humorous.' Mrs Warner 'put it all down' to her 'good mother and father – a good beginning in life', as did Mr Adams, aged 101.

There were a few mavericks who, in Mr Spinner's words 'contradicted all conventions in eating – I had a mother who believed in grocer's bills not doctor's bills'. Or in drinking – Mr Compton, an ex-sailor, according to his daughter, had 'rum instead of blood in his veins. He drinks alcohol like lemonade, given half a chance, though I've never seen him drunk.' He himself, in answer to the question said that he had 'just lived an ordinary life. I always said a prayer and thanked God for the well-being of myself and family and for safe return every time I went to sea.'

SUMMARY

In this chapter we have taken further the argument that very old people as a group cannot be seen as a typical cross section of the general population from which they are drawn. Here, it is as survivors that they display important characteristics which distinguish them. These features express the interaction of biographical influences, particularly family background and personal experiences, with the historical influences of a changing social structure.

It is impossible to predict in advance which individuals will survive into the tenth decade and beyond. Nevertheless, the impact of sex, social class and the age of parents all seem to play a significant part in affecting the chances of doing so. The impact of life style in promoting longevity is much more difficult to comment on though its effects in the future may well be considerable.

The themes of similarity and difference, both amongst our study group and between them and other groups in the population, will be further explored in subsequent chapters. We now turn to one of the most important issues in this respect – one which has a major impact on the quality of life – the health of the very old.

4

HEALTH AND DISABILITY

DEFINITIONS OF HEALTH

Despite the fact that health is at the centre of life's experience, it remains an elusive concept, more easily defined negatively, as the absence of disease, than positively. While the concept of health has an absolute ring to it – we all seem to know what it means even if we cannot quite say what it is – it also changes with circumstances and, most importantly, with age. The social meanings attached to health in childhood, in middle age and in old age, vary considerably. Expectations alter with changing phases of the life course. What would not be tolerated in earlier life may be accepted with the passing of the years, though this assumption needs careful scrutiny.

In general terms, health may be seen as a capacity, or resource, with which to carry out normal social roles, or as the successful adaptation to the physical and social environment. Parsons' (1951) early formulation of this concept of health drew attention to its social as well as its biological character. It is when the individual can no longer carry out social tasks and roles, and when the accommodation between the individual and the environment breaks down, that we speak of ill health in any socially significant sense (Zola 1966).

From this viewpoint, the presence of symptoms or physical limitations, by themselves, do not constitute ill-health. It is when they interfere with valued activities and goals that they become significant. It is this sociological aspect of health that helps us to understand the frequent discrepancy, to be found not least among the elderly, between the presence of symptoms and an individual's positive assessment of his or her own health. As has often been shown, people with considerable disabling conditions may continue to define themselves as healthy (Anderson and Bury 1988).

Part of the problem stems from the unavoidable reality that concepts such as disability are, by definition, somewhat arbitrary. Whilst it may be possible to assert that disease is either present or absent (for example, by recourse to specific laboratory tests) this is not possible with disability. This is because disability is a matter of degree and severity, not simply a matter of whether it is present or absent. So, for example, a recent survey of disability in Britain (Martin *et al.* 1988) depicted the range of disabilities and their severity in terms of levels of activity restriction. At the lower end of the scale, the 'threshold' under which an individual would be categorized as 'disabled' was based on the judgements of a panel of experts and lay people.

The survey found that over the age of 75, disability was more likely to be present than not (ibid: 18–21). Furthermore, a recent study by O'Connor *et al.* (1989) of nonagenarians found no-one in their sample to be without some form of significant physical or mental disability or illness.

In this way, expanding our definitions of health to take into account an ever-wider set of problems threatens to overwhelm us with the image of life, especially later life, as being characterized by compromised health. Whilst it is important, as a number of commentators have recently argued, that unmet health needs amongst the elderly, as in any other age group, are not accepted (or 'discounted') as a normal feature of ageing (Kalache *et al.* 1988; Martin *et al.* 1988), it is also important to bear in mind that subjective evaluations may not coincide with those held by professionals.

In this chapter, therefore, we attempt to give expression to the tension between an assessment of health which draws attention to the presence of illness and disability and one which takes into account the individual's evaluation of his or her own health status. In doing so we also extend our analysis of the common elements of experience in very old age, as well as the diversity and variability in such experiences.

We first describe the current health status of very old people in terms of chronic illness and disability (including the prevalence of pain and incontinence) and, briefly, mental illness. Following this we consider the evaluations of their health as seen by the respondents themselves.

PRESENT HEALTH STATUS

Chronic conditions

There is evidence elsewhere to show that ill-health does increase with age (see e.g. Victor 1987: 249, 250), though it is also argued that there is no justification for 'the popular stereotype of old age as a time of universal and inevitable chronic ill-health and impaired activity' (ibid). Comparisons with other studies present difficulties because of dissimilar age groups, the use of different measures, and variations in context. Allowing for these differences, the basic findings on the prevalence of chronic conditions among our sample fall mid-way between combined OPCS and GHS data showing relatively low levels of disability in very old age (ibid: 249) and the findings of two inner-city studies which showed high levels (Bowling *et al.* 1988: 28; Holme and Maizels 1990).

Seven per cent of the total sample said that they had no chronic conditions of any severity (see Appendix 2, Table A2.8). In this small group there were proportionately more men than women. We also found marginally fewer living in communal establishments than in their own homes in a ratio of five to three. The general health of the whole group reporting no chronic conditions was for the most part confirmed by the interviewers as 'good' or 'excellent'; in Mr Docker's case it was 'reasonable'. He was aged 91, was very active – going out regularly, and lived alone, with visits from his daughter almost every day and a chiropodist occasionally.

Mrs Brander, aged 93, lived in a residential home. She was described by the interviewer as 'tall, upright and bright, with good morale and excellent mental abilities'. Mrs Hetherington, aged 96, on the other hand, though able to perform almost all daily activities without difficulty, was nevertheless housebound.

At the other end of the scale, 14 per cent of our total sample members reported that they had five or more long-standing health problems, noticeably more so among the women. This was a lower proportion than found in Brent (Holme and Maizels 1990) and in City and Hackney (Bowling *et al.* 1988), where the lower age limits were 75 and 85, respectively. This may be simply a reflection of the fact that the elderly people of these other studies, unlike ours, were exclusively confined to inner-city areas. It was no surprise to find that the proportions in the two main types of residence were the converse of those where there were no chronic conditions – a ratio of two in communal establishments to one in private households.

The number of chronic conditions forms only a partial guide to state of health, and a somewhat crude one at that. To develop the point we must look to see what, in the main, they were suffering from – then how severe, in self-reported terms, the conditions were.

For the analysis we used a modified version of a GHS list of chronic

Table 4.1 Prevalence of main chronic conditions, excluding mental disorders: weighted sample

Chronic conditions	None or slight %	Rel. severe %	Very severe %	Total incap. %	Total subjects n=183–199 %
Blood pressure	92.1	6.5	1.4	0.0	100
Stroke	91.9	2.8	5.3	0.0	100
Trouble with legs	90.1	5.9	4.0	0.0	100
Heart	85.9	12.7	1.4	0.0	100
Lungs	80.0	16.1	3.9	0.0	100
Constipation	74.4	18.9	6.7	0.0	100
Sight	52.3	22.7	23.4	1.6	100
Arthritis, rheumatism	51.2	31.5	17.3	0.0	100
Hearing	48.1	29.9	18.6	3.4	100

disorders (OPCS 1977), focusing on ten conditions, which we thought would be most in evidence, and allowing for the noting of any others. As can be seen from Table 4.1, each condition has been recorded by its degree of severity. Unlike the highly complex measures of disability severity devised for the OPCS disability study (Martin *et al.* 1988), ours were based mainly on the self-reporting of the elderly people or, where necessary, on the opinion of proxy, carer and occasionally, where appropriate, interviewer.

We were particularly concerned to document the extent of trouble with eyesight and hearing amongst this group, as it turned out, with good reason. Of all the physical conditions mentioned by the study group, only eyesight and hearing were reported as causing 'total incapacity'; one woman and five men belonging to the actual sample in the former case, and six women and one man in the latter. In addition, 46 per cent of the total sample reported 'relatively severe' or 'severe' trouble with their eyes, and even more, 49 per cent, with their hearing. Thus, over half the sample, including all but one of those over the age of 100, had serious trouble with deafness. For men in particular, as with Mr Hitchcock, deafness may well have preceded old age as a result of occupational and other hazards, though as far as prevalence was concerned there were no very marked sex differences.

As far as we could tell, of the thirty-three members of the actual sample with 'very severe' deafness only a quarter were apparently using an aid and, among those whose deafness was described as 'relatively severe' (forty-nine), the figure was only one-fifth. Mrs James had apparently lent her hearing aid to 'someone in the kitchen' of her residential home and had not had it back, but in any case, it seems, 'it didn't do much good'. Judging from our taped interviews, very few reaped much advantage from them. This is in line with other research (see e.g. Wenger 1988: 22).

From the carer's point of view, severe deafness can prove to be a formidable drain on patience and the capacity to care. And, of course, the afflicted person can suffer great loneliness and a sense of isolation. Such conditions can lead to a withdrawal from social interaction and a rise in feelings of embarrassment and stigma (Strauss 1975).

One of the five blind men, 96-year-old Mr Compton, exemplified particularly the stereotype of blindness cheerfully borne. Living in harmony with a devoted 54-year-old daughter, her husband and two teenage children, he was 'always glad to get up and eager to find out what's happening outside'. Not far short of half of those with relatively poor eyesight were unable to go out. Nevertheless, of those who did, nearly one-third could do so alone, the majority 'without difficulty'. Furthermore, four out of the five with very poor eyesight who went out alone did so, they claimed, without difficulty. This independence was further illustrated by the fact that over half the total partially-sighted sample lived alone.

All the women and men, with one exception, suffering from five or more chronic conditions had hearing trouble – mostly of great severity. Mrs Storace, aged 91, was the exception; she also had good eyesight, unlike the great majority of this group with multiple conditions. Her problems consisted of a heart condition, arthritis, a chest condition, high blood pressure and 'agitation', all scored as 'relatively severe'. She was confined to her residential home but within those limits was active and cheerful and described by the owner of the home as a 'strong-minded character with a strong constitution. She is a World War I widow who had to cope alone.' Mrs Storace herself reckoned that she had no energy but described her fitness as 'fair'.

In between the two extremes of frailty as defined by the presence of multiple chronic disorders, or their complete absence, were the great majority of the sample with from one to four reported long-standing health problems of varying degrees of severity. But, whether belonging to either of the extreme groups, or to the middle one, the few examples we have given already highlight the complexities involved in assessing health status amongst the very old.

Arthritis, the scourge of the elderly, particularly women, certainly took its toll among our sample, nearly half of whom were afflicted, echoing the findings of Wenger (1988: 13) and of Bowling et al. (1988: 29) where the prevalence was even greater. Over half the women in our sample reported a severe, or relatively severe, condition. Mrs Cuthbert, living in a residential home, was severely limited by her arthritis in her mobility and her ability to perform many daily activities, yet was cheerful and uncomplaining. 'Yes', she told the interviewer, 'I do have a lot of pain – in my joints and when I walk [she used a frame], but I manage and I always have my visitors to look forward to.' Mrs Locke, by contrast, was 'fed up', saying further, 'I want to die'.

A very small proportion of the sample – just under 2 per cent – were, it seems, suffering from a very severe heart condition, with a further 13 per cent placing themselves in the 'relatively severe' category. A 93-year-old widower, when asked if his heart was a problem, replied amidst great chuckling 'not from the health point of view'. Since a third of the sample were apparently taking a diuretic, it is fair to assume that a further group had a mild heart condition. Even smaller proportions - mainly the younger women – were suffering from the aftermath of strokes, or 'trouble with legs', often a common complaint among the elderly. Some form of lung or chest condition afflicted one-fifth of the sample.

We should add that constipation troubled one-quarter of the total sample. Diabetes, anaemia, dizziness in the morning, stomach disorders affected four or five members of the actual sample; eight (all, bar one, male) mentioned hernia, and seven were described by their proxies or interviewers as generally, and extremely, frail. At least five female members of the actual sample were still suffering from the aftermath of the serious injury most often associated with old age in women – a broken femur.

The prevalence of these conditions is partially reflected in the number of times elderly people are admitted to hospital. Of the total sample, nearly half had not been admitted at all during the past five years. Of the remainder, the majority had been in once.

A further indication of health status in this connection may, if somewhat crudely, be gleaned from the fact that nearly three-quarters of the sample were taking a wide range of preparations (on average about two per person), though the minority – more than one-quarter – who took nothing is an important one. These preparations did not include pain-killers or sedatives.

Pain

Pain is an almost inevitable corollary of swollen joints and damaged bones, muscles and nerves arising from rheumatic or arthritic conditions. Other physical disorders suffered by the sample also caused pain or, at the least, discomfort. Though the effective use of painkillers will obviously mitigate some of the consequences of pain, it must, in any of its manifestations, adversely affect the quality of life. It is in this context, therefore, that we shall later return to the subject. Meanwhile, what proportion of the sample did complain of pain or discomfort?

Here it is advisable to consider the actual sample as represented in the four different sex/age groups, for there are some important differences between them (see Appendix 2, Table A2.9). Thus, among the men, half the 90–94 year age group complained of pain or discomfort and slightly fewer of the older age group. The older group of women was apparently the least affected, though there were still as many as two-fifths. It was, however, among the younger women that pain or discomfort figured most – over seven in ten of the forty-two replying. These differences may reflect the particularly robust character of some of our very oldest survivors.

There are a variety of ways in which pain may be assessed; so we asked a series of questions, which included the request to describe the pain in their own words. These resolved themselves into three main categories: when the pain occurred; where it occurred; what type of pain it was. Only 13 per cent of those suffering pain or discomfort described it as constant. For half, it came at night and for one-third when they were standing. Walking caused pain for just under half and changing position for just over half.

Understandably, people seemed to find it difficult to locate exactly the site of their pain, but just over a third talked of their head or limbs while only 8 per cent said that their whole body ached. The type of pain also was not easily described. For 7 per cent it was quite simply 'horrible'. 'Pulling', 'sharp', 'an ache', 'throbbing' were terms variously used by small proportions.

All in all we gained the impression that pain was not a dominant factor in most people's lives, though a few individuals suffered constant pain. No doubt the fact that two-fifths of the sample were taking painkillers not only alleviated the pain but may well have masked some of its features.

Sleep

Sleep patterns may vary from one person to another, or, for the same person, from one period of the life course to another, for physiological or psychological reasons or both. Changes may occur with age; 'bad' or 'good' sleep may be persistent or sporadic; people's sleep 'needs' vary. In old age sleeping at night may be particularly affected by the tendency to sleep in the day. All of which means that sleep is difficult to use as a health indicator.

Nevertheless, constant trouble with sleep can be debilitating and depressing so we asked the members of the sample whether they had recently had any trouble sleeping. Something under two-thirds said that they never had; a handful did have trouble but this was nothing new, while, for the remaining group (nearly one-third), poor sleep was a relatively recent experience. It was among the younger women that the proportions were highest in both these last categories.

Among the population at large, particularly among women, there has recently been considerable debate in Britain about tranquillizer use and dependence, including those drugs used to induce sleep (Gabe and Bury 1988). Among our sample, the proportions who regularly took something to help them sleep (proportionately, but only marginally, more women than men) were relatively low – one-quarter – and as many as two-thirds of the sample never took anything.

It is interesting to note that of the eleven individuals who said they were in constant pain, only four took a sedative (three did not reply to this question), all to good effect. Of the four who did not take anything, Mrs Plater slept, apparently, 'like a top', Mrs Nisbett always read in bed for half an hour and had 'no trouble', but Mrs Trevor and Mrs Holland had sleep problems – difficulty falling asleep and lying awake for long periods. Mr Matthews, when asked if he took anything to help him sleep, replied with a chuckle, 'Just my wife; I take her to bed.'

Incontinence

Among those who have reached, or contemplate, old age, probably one of the conditions most dreaded is that of incontinence. Stories of neglect and distress in nursing homes and residential homes abound, not only from journalistic investigation (see e.g. Yorkshire Television 1987; Hicks 1988) but also from more rigorous studies (e.g. Hughes and Wilkin 1987). In the community, family carers are reported in a number of studies as being frequently involved in the desolating task of tending and cleaning up the incontinent, often with little support from the formal services (Anderson 1988).

Such accounts, and the implications they carry for both individuals and carer, are certainly not exaggerated though, by the media, the emphasis may be. It must, however, be said that among very old people the prevalence of incontinence appears to be less than might commonly be supposed. Eighty per cent of our total sample reported no urinary incontinence and 85 per cent no trouble with their bowels. There were no marked differences between men and women.

There were, however, decided differences according to where the elderly people were living (see Appendix 2, Tables A2.10 and A2.11). Thus, 91 per cent of those in private households were fully continent, and sufferers from daily incontinence in either form were to be found almost exclusively in communal establishments – predominantly hospitals and nursing homes. Mrs Preston, for example, whom we met earlier, was one. The onset of this affliction, coupled with a series of falls, had precipitated the move away from her son and daughter-in-law. Still visiting every day, they had been 'very upset' when she had to go into hospital even though looking after her 'had created a lot of worry and a lot of work'.

Mobility

Turning from the various chronic conditions we have so far discussed, the degree of mobility, or what the OPCS study researchers have categorized as locomotion (Martin *et al.* 1988), is an important starting point in assessing the extent of disability. As can be seen from Table 4.2, 59 per cent of the total sample reported that they never went out. Of these, approximately one-tenth were confined to their beds.

Within each sex group there were expected age differences in that the older women and men, particularly the women and particularly those over the age of 100, were less mobile than the younger. But apparent also were significant sex differences, as found in other studies (see e.g. Victor 1987: 250). Fifty-five per cent of the men, for example, could go out compared with 38 per cent of the women; twice as many women as men needed help within doors. A large part of these differences is accounted for by the presence of arthritis in women. A significantly higher proportion of women were bedbound.

It is important to note that only 52 per cent of the domiciliary-based sample were totally housebound, compared with 66 per cent of those in

Table 4.2 Degrees of mobility be sex: weighted sample

	Women %	Men %	Total %	
Bedbound	7.8	2.5	6.7	⎫
Housebound, needing help	32.5	32.5	19.5	⎬ 58.8
Housebound, no help needed	22.0	10.0	32.6	⎭
Can go out with help	27.9	47.5	9.4	⎫ 41.2
Can go out without help	9.7	7.5	31.8	⎭
Total	100[1]	100	100	
	(154)	(40)	(194)	

[1]See note 2.

communal establishments. Over three-fifths of all the housebound living in private households (excluding the bedbound) said that they needed no help to move about within doors, though, as we shall see, many did need help for other activities.

Returning to the total sample of those who could go out, the majority did so regularly, about half of these on a daily basis. 'Going out', as we shall see in later chapters, combines several factors including physical strength, confidence and a sense of safety, and, of course, a reason for venturing forth. Confidence and physical strength may be partially measured by the extent to which very old people use public transport. This is quickly dealt with. It comes, perhaps, as no surprise that the vast majority of the sample members – 96 per cent – were unable or unwilling to use public transport. Whether this proportion would be smaller if more attention were paid to the needs of elderly people *vis à vis* their means of outdoor locomotion (see e.g. Age Concern, England 1978) and the physical restrictions of the outside environment for the disabled (Buchanan and Chamberlain 1978) is difficult to say.

The gender differences generally in mobility were further in evidence in the nature of their expeditions. Four of the men, for instance, and no women were car drivers, though one woman had, it seems, driven her car until the age of 88. Over three-fifths of the women never went for a walk compared with two-fifths of the men. Similar, more marked, differences are apparent with shopping expeditions and to a lesser extent with attendance at clubs.

Being housebound expresses both physical limitations and social constraints (Barker and Bury 1978). In the presence of poor health or disability, outdoor activities may seem to be more trouble than they are worth. But this does not mean that being housebound is a clear measure of functional limitation or, alternatively, that people would not choose to go out if circumstances were different. What it does show is that mobility and valued activities interact in complex ways. Individuals make strategic decisions about the value of remaining mobile or going out compared with the desire to reduce risk and remain safe by staying at home.

Activities of daily living

By their presence or absence, the various kinds of physical conditions we have so far discussed will all in one way or another affect the elderly person's ability to perform certain tasks. This task-based approach to disability has been summarized in indices of 'activities of daily living' (ADLs). Many of these might seem to be fundamental to daily life, such as dressing, washing, climbing stairs and the like. Yet, as we noted at the beginning of this chapter, disability is a 'slippery' concept (Topliss 1975:20). Some activities, for example, may no longer be relevant in a changed environment. The ability to climb stairs means little if the individual has moved to a bungalow, and even dressing may be facilitated by a series of adaptations such as the use of zips instead of difficult buttons.

Furthermore, tasks frequently touch on role performance. In other words the ability or inability to carry out ADLs may touch on aspects of the person as a whole, by creating, for example, dependence on another for help. The need for such help can rarely be given or received without the relationship being affected. In this case we move from dealing with disability to that of handicap, which focuses on the disadvantage caused by the consequences of poor task and role performance.

Using a modified list of activities of daily living and again relying primarily on self-reports, supplemented by those of proxies or carers, we attempted to scale the ADLs of sample members on a 'can do' basis: on four points from 'can easily' to 'cannot'. Table 4.3 shows the results for the total sample.

If we look at the table from the top down we find a relatively large proportion of the sample who were able to perform three of the basic functions of daily living – feeding themselves, washing their face and hands and combing their hair or shaving. As many as 29 per cent needed help in using the toilet and 43 per cent were unable to dress themselves

Table 4.3 Activities of daily living: weighted sample

Activities	Easy	Difficult		Cannot	Total
		alone	with help		subjects n=177–199
	%	%	%	%	%
Feeding self	71.2	10.4	14.0	4.4	100[1]
Washing face and hands	64.5	10.9	12.7	12.0	100
Combing hair/shaving	61.6	11.0	7.5	19.9	100
Using toilet	56.5	14.4	13.7	15.3	100
Dressing self	39.9	17.0	22.1	21.0	100
Writing letters	30.1	7.2	4.2	58.5	100
Fiddly jobs	26.0	7.1	3.3	63.6	100
Light household jobs	25.9	13.6	3.3	57.2	100
Bathing self	22.7	7.0	35.7	34.6	100
Preparing a meal	21.7	10.3	5.4	62.7	100
Negotiating steps	20.5	22.3	23.4	33.8	100
Negotiating stairs	17.1	18.3	15.0	49.7	100
Cutting toe nails	11.6	5.3	4.9	78.3	100

[1]See note 2.

without some help. Thereafter the proportions in the 'easy' category fall consistently until we find that only 12 per cent were able to cut their toe nails. Insignificant though this last task may seem, it must be done, and has considerable bearing on the ability to move about.

Table 4.3. shows that only 35 per cent of the sample were able to negotiate stairs without help, an indication of the presence of considerable physical limitations, though, as we have suggested, much depends on the need to use stairs and the availability of alternative living arrangements. There were among the sample, examples where some adaptations had been made and others where they were noticeable by their absence. But adaptations may also increase difficulties in other areas of life, as when, for example, a bed is moved to a downstairs room thereby crowding the living space for others in the household.

One way of developing our understanding of disability among the sample members is to move beyond treating each activity separately (as we have done in Table 4.3) and to compute an overall disability score which can be used to summarize the position of individuals or subgroups. By combining all items scored as either 'difficult' or 'cannot', as we have done, we have constructed a 'percentage disability score' (PDS) (see note 4). This exercise has to be regarded with some caution in that we have combined items that might have different implications for daily life, but it does allow us to make some more general comments concerning disability among our study members.

The differences, for example, between men and women which we have already described are underlined when we look at their scores. The mean PDS for the group as a whole is 55 per cent, with women scoring on average 57 per cent and men 47 per cent, the difference being statistically significant.

We have seen that with the earlier health-status measures of chronic illness and, especially, mobility there were differences in prevalence or performance according to the two main types of residence. Here with ADLs, significant differences between the two groups were apparent (see Appendix 2, Table A2.12). Invariably, those in communal establishments were more likely than those in private households to be unable to perform the listed activities unaided. In three instances – feeding themselves, washing face and hands or going to the toilet, proportionately over four times as many of the former group were in this category.

These differences between private households and communal establishments are particularly underlined if we use percentage disability scores. Remembering that the mean score for the whole group is 55 per cent, those in private households scored on average 43 per cent and those in communal establishments an average of 68 per cent. This suggests that an increase in the level of disability is associated with entering a communal establishment, though some individuals may suffer an increase in disability having made such a move. The complexities of the relationship between disability and the environment are perhaps best illustrated by a particular example.

Mrs Horden lived on her own in a housing-association flat. She suffered from poor eyesight, relatively severe deafness and arthritis, and said that she had a weak chest. Despite these problems she was able to go out and had, by our calculations, a low level of disability. She recounted the following unhappy incident.

> I can't get down in the bath. I've got a shower and I stand up in the bath. I got caught in there one night and I was there about an hour. I let the water out and I couldn't turn round – it's a narrow bath and eventually I put a towel at the bottom of the bath to stand on and of course that was wet too and I slid all over the show. The only way I managed to get out was by grabbing the wash basin but I was frozen stiff. I wouldn't try again after that –

it frightened me. It was when I was going to bed at half past ten at night and I couldn't call anybody as it's all locked up. We've got an emergency cord that shows a light outside. It's supposed to be connected to Dr Dixon who is next door, but they're never there. It would be left to anyone passing. Later the Red Cross brought a seat but it goes right across the top – I'd be perched up, so I don't use it.

This illustration demonstrates a number of points: independence spiked with apprehension, and resulting in near disaster; failure of a system of supervision; an ill-considered attempt at a solution with the provision of an aid remaining unused, a situation unfortunately all too common; an unsatisfactory resolution (ceasing to shower), all of which added up to the creation of substantial disadvantage or handicap rather than disability as such.

Mental illness

So far we have considered mainly physical disability. Here we turn to mental health problems. For the purpose of this study we have grouped under this heading two main conditions: the range of impairment from mild confusion to dementia and various degrees of depression.

On the basis of the proxies' replies, the carers' assessments and the interviewers' observations, 5 per cent of the total sample were deemed to have dementia. The *actual* numbers comprised six women of whom five were aged over 95, and five men, of whom one was in the older age group. This is not to say that serious, or quite serious, confusion or memory loss, acute enough to warrant a proxy or part-proxy interview (noticeably so among the centenarians), was not evident among others who were interviewed. In fact, of the total sample, a further 14 per cent were suffering from confusion or memory loss, and here the proportion among younger women was markedly the highest. Then there were a few other individuals, noted by the interviewers, and evident from the taped interviews, who had 'lapses of memory', or 'slight confusion', most of whom managed well enough to give a reasonably reliable interview – though with inevitable gaps – on their own.

So, according to these findings, the stereotype of a *majority* group of senile, dependent people, once extreme old age is reached, does not hold, though we do not wish to underplay the fact of memory loss or mild confusion, nor to underestimate the impact of dementia or serious confusion on the individual's quality of life. Neither, for the minority living in private households, do we underrate the implications for the carer, particularly as many among this minority group, also had high levels of disability.

Depression

Here again we relied wherever possible on the elderly people's own assessment of any depressive tendencies they may have had, though drawing on other research (see Appendix 1, section 9) to give a framework to the subject. One question asked if they had been under the doctor at all for nerves or depression. Of the total sample replying, just under one-fifth replied in the affirmative, but for only half of these was it within the previous five years.

A relatively positive picture also emerged from a series of questions about the state of their spirits in the past week. As many as 53 per cent said these had been good and a further 17 per cent excellent; for 9 per cent spirits had been 'mixed'; which leaves 18 per cent of the sample who had been feeling 'low' and 3 per cent 'very depressed'. The older women, on the whole, seemed most likely to have been in low spirits and the younger men least likely.

Moreover, only a minority of the total sample – 34 per cent (more proportionately among the women than the men) – said that they easily became upset or irritable. 'What can't be cured must be endured' was Mrs Stead's maxim, while Mr Crawford told the interviewer that he never got upset because, along with Wordsworth, he had 'felt the presence of elevated thoughts'.

Among those who had had recent or past experiences of depression or low spirits, only two – one woman and one man both over 95 – had ever felt 'suicidal'. Mr Abbott revealed his feelings:

> If I tell you I was the life and soul of any party that I was connected with and I don't even laugh at anything now, you'll know how I've changed. I get very depressed. Suicidal? Yes, that's just how I feel. I have felt that if I were brave enough I would do away with myself but I have always felt the fear of pain.

Two younger women and three men (two in the younger age group) felt 'hopeless', and ten, mostly younger, women and four younger men felt 'weepy'. But for the majority of this group their overall mood was 'not too bad'; they could 'usually snap out of it'. These various self-

Table 4.4 Self-perceptions of fitness: weighted sample

Degree of fitness	%
Very unfit	3.3
Unfit	4.7
Fair	47.3
Good	26.0
Excellent	18.7
Total	100
	(150)

assessments were, on the whole, in line with those of the interviewers and carers.

All that we have discussed hitherto in this chapter, though based on self-reports, possesses an 'objective' descriptive element, in that it has been concerned with conditions or prevalence or performance. We now turn to the purely subjective matter of feelings.

HEALTH STATUS AND SUBJECTIVE FEELINGS

Views were sought on three main topics: how fit they felt; how much energy they had; how they thought their health compared with others of their own age.

Replies to the first two questions showed, on the whole, a positive and optimistic response. As can be seen in Table 4.4, only 8 per cent of the total sample replying said they were unfit or very unfit and, at the other end of the scale, 45 per cent said their health was good or excellent, with 47 per cent rating it as 'fair'. Similarly, over half the sample said that they had a 'fair amount' of energy or 'a lot'. Interestingly, there was very little difference of view between men and women in their fitness assessments, and, with energy, the younger women gave a slightly more favourable account than their male counterparts.

Yet these self-assessments bear only a limited relation to elderly people's physical condition as reported by themselves, or to their ability to perform various tasks. Just over half those who placed themselves on the two highest points of the fitness scale said they could not go out or prepare a meal on their own. Light domestic jobs were impossible for half those rating their health as 'excellent' and a similar proportion of the same group were either unable to negotiate stairs alone or needed help. Such examples can be multiplied and illustrate the desire of elderly people, already referred to, to maintain a healthy image (see also Bond 1987: 473–76), though, unusually, one recent study has found that the elderly were less optimistic in their subjective evaluations than the middle-aged (ibid).

It must also be said, whether justifiably or not, that to be 'fit' in extreme old age carries different connotations from fitness at earlier ages. The authors (Levkoff *et al.* 1986) of one of the studies referred to by Bond (1987: 474) suggest that 'if older people do report more health optimism, it must be only when asked to compare themselves with their age peers'. In our study, such optimism, as we have seen in the sample members' response to the fitness and energy questions, did not have to rely on comparisons. Optimism, however, was evident at an even higher rate in response to a question inviting comparison. Eighty per cent of the total sample replying considered that they had better health than others of the same age. Mr Unwin, for example, spoke for many with his reply, 'When I see them wheeled about in wheel chairs and God knows what and staggering along with crutches, it seems to me that I am not too bad, perhaps'.

SUMMARY

In this chapter we have described the health of a sample of people aged 90 and over in England today. This profile expresses, we feel, many of the tensions that are inherent in survival into very old age. Whilst we have shown that life after 90 is associated with high risks of disability and failing powers, more generally, such survival must also involve avoiding or weathering many a health storm. This is especially the case for men, and for those from working-class backgrounds, who may have survived very much against the odds.

Even the presence of disability or chronic illness may not always mean the end of valued activities or a reasonable life style. Adaptations over long periods of time might mitigate the effects of disability, but this makes it difficult to interpret findings, including our own, which show reduced functioning. Such findings may be due to a reduction in activity alone or a change in outlook, or, of course, a complex interaction of both, across the later part of the life course. They direct our attention to the *importance* of daily activities to the individual, and to the value they place upon them, as much as to the *ability* to do them. The tension between these facets of experience may help to explain many of the discrepancies between objective and subjective measures.

Moreover, we have also seen that the health of those over 90 years of age contains much variation. We have seen individuals still very active and others leading a more sedentary life. A smaller group are facing serious health problems, many of them, perhaps, as they come towards the end of their very long lives. These findings underline the diversity of experience among the oldest old and our contention that very old age is not a uniform process of decline.

At the same time we are mindful of the need to recognize health needs where they are in evidence, and especially where they might affect carers if not the individual. We have no wish to paint an overly optimistic picture, or 'discount' the effects of poor health or disability because of age itself. Adaptation, and changed expectations may be functional for the individual, but they may also mask real needs which could be met. Certainly the frequency with which we encountered serious levels of sensory impairments, and overall high levels of disability, especially as the result of arthritis in women, underlines the presence of considerable health-related problems amongst those aged 90 and over.

One way, however, of developing our understanding of health amongst the very old is to place it within the wider context of quality of life, alongside other experiences and values. It is, therefore, to this broader concept of the quality of life that we now turn.

5

THE QUALITY OF LIFE

In the lives of the very old, as in the lives of people at all stages of the life course, material circumstances and health are central to the quality of life. Without an adequate level of both (defined within the context of prevailing values), the pleasure of living, it is held, is likely to diminish. With a poor level of both, living can turn into mere existence. It is not surprising, therefore, that much public discussion (and today, of course, media coverage) concerns itself with the needs of the elderly, or those of other vulnerable age-related groups, such as deprived children.

Such public discussion rehearses our worst fears and reassures us that the problems are being tackled. In this way the 'needs of strangers' (Ignatieff 1987) are taken care of while we continue pursuing our own interests and projects. Thus it is possible to find research evidence which shows the persistence of collectivist beliefs in the welfare state and the care of those in need (West et al. 1984) at a time when voting patterns have favoured policies which reduce public expenditure and lower taxation. To say the least, 'dependent groups' exist in social circumstances of some ambiguity.

Our own discussion, so far, has covered ground similar to many social surveys on needs and circumstance, albeit amongst a group of elderly people that has received little attention in the literature. Yet there are at least two reasons to be cautious about relying on our evidence so far as giving a sufficient picture of the quality of life in very old age. First, while common sense dictates that adequate housing, income and health are essential conditions of life, it is less clear how they influence its quality. The *processes* which transform resources available to the individual, such as income, into satisfying experiences are less than clear cut, and need to be studied in their own right.

Secondly, questions might be asked about the impact of health on the life course and on everyday life, particularly in today's cultural climate, where improving or promoting health has taken on an almost religious character. The purpose of health promotion has become almost self-evident, even though we know little about how it actually affects the quality of life. As we pointed out earlier in this book, little is known about the effects of health promotion on the quality of life of the very old, and its attempts to reduce the commonly regarded 'risk factor' (Brody 1985; Patrick 1986).

By the same token, while common sense dictates that the relatively high levels of disability shown in the last chapter are bound to have negative consequences for the individual, whether this is as the direct result of reduced functioning, or the impact of disability on the individual's self-concept and interactional skills, remains to be examined. Though concepts such as disability and handicap complement traditional concepts of health status based on disease and illness, even these must be extended into broader considerations of well-being if they are adequately to capture the nature of contemporary experience, especially for the survivors into very old age. There are differences between our exploration of *can do* and *do do* and *want to do* in the area of daily activities, and these may be explained by changing *expectations* across the life course and between different groups.

In order to arrive at a fuller picture of the lives of the very old, we need to know what *meanings* are attached to both material circumstances and health, and how they fit in with other valued areas of life. Only in this way will we be able to avoid a reductionist view of old age. This much has already emerged from our discussion, but it can be emphasized by turning to the wider perspective of quality of life. As indicated, there is a need to supplement a concern with material circumstances and health with a broader perspective that draws on concepts of psychological and social 'well-being'. In this way, an overly medicalized and self-evident view of old age can be resisted, and the values, perceptions and expectations of the individuals, their peers and their families can be brought into view. These processes 'mediate' objective circumstances and help us understand why, for example, older people may appear to be less distressed by chronic illness than those in younger age groups (Cassileth *et al.* 1984).

This chapter, then, acts as a bridge between our earlier discussion of health and material circumstances and these wider considerations. In order to serve this purpose we offer an initial definition of quality of life in the context of old age and then discuss some of the reasons for the growing importance of the concept and its application in the research literature. Having done this we can then examine, in more detail in the chapters which follow, the application of quality-of-life measures in the context of very old age and our own study.

DEFINING THE CONCEPT

Of all the discussions of quality of life and the elderly currently available, George and Bearon's (1980) influential résumé is perhaps the most useful for our purposes. In their discussion, they recognize the difficulties of definition but attempt to bring together the two main sets of factors: objective conditions and subjective evaluations.

'Objective conditions' refer to the assets (we might say, resources) which people can call on to deal with life's challenges, particularly their health and their financial security. Despite all their present complexity in the context of the very old, they are clearly central to the quality of life assessment. 'Subjective evaluations' refers to a range of life experiences, and includes: 'perceptions of well-being, a basic level of satisfaction or contentment, and a general sense of self-worth' (ibid: 2).

This dual concept, which includes 'the conditions of life and the experience of life' (ibid), may be put more schematically, thus:

DIMENSIONS OF QUALITY OF LIFE

Objective conditions

General health and functional status
Socio-economic status

Subjective evaluations

Life satisfaction and related measures
Self-esteem and related measures

The four dimensions under the two broad headings reflect, for George and Bearon (ibid: 6), central values in contemporary American society (see also Parsons (1951) for an early discussion of the place of health within the American value system). But they are also relevant, in our view, to the English context. A brief comment on each of the four dimensions might help to clarify this point.

Taking health and functional status first, George and Bearon (op.cit.) comment that although these are capable of being defined by

84

professionally derived norms, subjective ratings can equally well be used. In our discussion of these in the last chapter, we gave special emphasis to functional status, as measured by activities of daily living. Our task now is therefore to bring these findings into the broader context of their impact on subjective experience and daily life. They can be placed against other valued areas of daily life, such as family support or social activities.

Similarly, material circumstances, however much they represent shared values (we all, for example, value the availability of proper heating arrangements or the supply of hot water in our homes), cannot be easily separated from subjective responses. What, for example, are we to make of the fact that some in our sample lived at home without proper heating or, indeed, an inside lavatory (one of the classic historical indicators of an inadequate 'material' quality of life) but did not express any dissatisfaction with such arrangements?

George and Bearon (1980) comment that there is, in general, an understandable presumption that material, especially financial assets, affect quality of life in later years. 'It is less clear, however, *precisely how* economic conditions contribute to life experience. For example, do financial assets operate such that the more one has the better one's life experience?' (ibid: 12). We think that questions such as these are particularly relevant to very old people, where perceptions of need may have been formed under very different historical conditions, and where they may have persisted or changed throughout a long life course. Under these circumstances perceptions and expectations may be different from those of other groups, for example, the 'young elderly'. Moreover, as discussed earlier, we are also obliged to consider the difference between direct and indirect effects, in that life style frequently 'mediates' objective circumstances. These comments do not, of course, imply that 'objective needs' may be 'discounted' because of changed expectations, but that perceptions held by the old person, the family and professional contacts are likely to contain discrepancies in outlook.

As far as the subjective dimensions of quality of life are concerned, these combine several measures concerning life satisfaction which can be summarized in two basic ways. Life satisfaction may be used as a general or 'global' measure of past, present or (anticipated) future states, and may be expressed in terms of happiness or a sense of well-being with life as a whole. Second, particularly with respect to residential arrangements and day-to-day experiences, including interpersonal relationships, it may be possible to link life satisfaction to specific aspects of experience, for example family interaction. Horley

(1984: 124) maintains that this latter domain of quality-of-life measures, including 'day-to-day specific action . . . has been virtually ignored to date'.

Measures of self-esteem, by contrast, direct our attention to social psychological components of experience. For George and Bearon (1980: 6) the essential evaluation here is of the self as an object and of judgements about the degree of success in 'personal interaction and negotiation with the environment'. At the social level, 'status attainment' through the life course may produce a sense of success or failure, (Riley *et al.* 1988) whereas satisfaction or dissatisfaction with relationships may have a particular influence on psychological status. In this way measures of well-being may be contrasted with psychological measures of self-worth.

The ability to negotiate change and to make effective choices, however, directs attention to the relative power held by individuals and their carers, as well as other significant individuals in the person's life. The increased reliance with age on formal services may run the risk of increasing feelings of being in need or dependent, or reinforce a sense of loss of role thus reducing self-esteem. George and Bearon (1980) make the point that there is frequently a set of delicate 'trade offs' to be made here, in opting for different kinds of living arrangements. Before we attempt to apply this conceptual framework, particularly its subjective dimensions, we highlight the broader historical circumstances that have given rise to quality-of-life research, and its application to the ageing field, in recent years. This will provide a useful context for considering our own use of the concept. It will also help us point out some of the pitfalls and difficulties in employing the concept.

THE RISE OF QUALITY-OF-LIFE MEASURES

Measures and their uses

As Najman and Levine (1981: 107) have argued, the development of quality-of-life measures has occurred within the context of post-war social development, characterized by 'an early interest in the use of objective social indicators as a form of social monitoring' (see also Carley 1981). Social and political debates about poverty and the distribution of resources increasingly required evidence and measures which allow comparison. Yet Najman and Levine (1980: 102) go on to argue that such objective measures 'have not been useful in guiding social policy'. Vagueness of definition and weakness of measurement are part of the problem. It is also now apparent that there has been a lack of fit between objective and subjective measures, of particular significance in old age and especially very old age. We have already discussed in the last chapter variations in the experience of health and disability from this viewpoint.

As a consequence, a potential gap has opened up between profession-ally derived norms for health and well-being and those held by particular groups in society. The discrepancy between 'lay beliefs' and scientifically defined norms requires careful investigation, especially where it can be shown that lay beliefs make a significant difference to the perception of problems and to the behaviour of individuals in the face of adversity. Blaxter (1976), for example, has shown that significant differences can arise between individuals' perceptions of disability and those held by administrators and doctors. Moreover, this 'clash of perspectives' (Freidson 1970) may help explain many of the differences that occur between, on the one hand, expectations by professionals (for example, in the take-up of services or compliance with treatment regimens) and, on the other, the 'cultural logic' of lay perceptions and actions (Mechanic 1968; Calnan 1987).

The history of research on subjective measures, however, has raised difficulties similar to those on objective measures. Horley, (1984) for example, discusses two main long-standing concerns: the lack of conceptual clarity and consistency in definitions, and the difference between overall assessments of life satisfaction and those of a more day-to-day kind, which we have already distinguished. In this way, current quality-of-life research may be seen as part of a long-standing concern with the complex 'study of adjustment in the aged', (ibid: 125) which stems from the work of researchers such as Havighurst (1951) in the 1940s and 1950s.

Reviews of these developments warn us against placing too much weight on quality-of-life research which purports to solve social- or health-policy issues, rather than being content with the more modest aim of using it to focus our attention on important aspects of experience. In particular, where measures are based on concepts that have a wide common-sense usage, we should not expect to achieve 'terminological invariance' which is often the basis for establishing valid and reliable indicators (Horley 1984: 126). In our own use, for example, of the term 'morale' we have relied on common-sense understanding rather than a technical definition.

In addition to the problems of definition and measurement, there is also a wider intellectual problem that should be raised at this point. Put simply, we must be aware of the danger of substituting for a reductionist 'medicalization' of old age, an even more pervasive form of surveillance based on social and psychological measures. We do not have to be conspiritorial to recognize that there are many claims to expertise in this area, by many professional groups and researchers with a variety of interests of their own. This alone should make us question the purposes and effects of quality-of-life research currently underway in gerontology, as in other social science fields.

Armstrong (1983) for example, has argued that post-war British developments of social techniques, including research methods such as the social survey, marked a shift in the nature of social order to include more subtle and elusive forms of social control. Coercive forms of power gave way to forms of authority based on ever-expanding professional expertise. Rather than being told how to behave, post-war populations have increasingly been asked for their opinions. The proliferation of opinion-poll research pays continuing testament to this process.

From this viewpoint, to focus on subjective meaning as opposed to objective measures is less a mark of social progress than a way of monitoring and thus ordering social life. Professional groups and their fields of expertise may be subtly (or not so subtly) informing and shaping experience, even as their clients' 'subjective' needs are monitored and met. The claim to welfare and concern which such research purports to embody may disguise current values which, if made explicit, would not necessarily prove universally acceptable. The emphasis on subjective meaning from this viewpoint disguises as much as it reveals.

We think that the expansion of the socio-medical 'gaze' to take in an ever-increasing number of objective and subjective indicators, does carry dangers of this sort. Indeed, we were only too aware of them as we set up our own research, in our identification of the 'very old' as an object of study. Yet we feel that the alleged negative aspects of modern social research can be greatly overstated (for a longer discussion of this issue in the context of medical sociology research, see Bury 1986). Whilst it is undoubtedly true that the elderly, and especially the very old, are 'at risk' in research of being portrayed in stereotypical ways that they may resent, as a 'burden', for example, or a 'challenge' (Wells and Freer 1988), this does not get round the fact that, in a more conventional sense, individuals or groups among the very old may be 'at risk' in terms of health and social needs (see Chapter 7 for a fuller discussion of 'risk'). We should certainly approach quality-of-life issues with caution and in a reflective way, but to offer nothing other than a 'critique' of such measures is, in our view, to evade many of the real problems of old age that exist in our communities, and the related need for research.

The growth and purpose of evaluation

There is one other contextual or historical factor to consider in connection with the development of quality-of-life research, namely the growth of evaluation. In most developed countries, the rapid post-war development of health and welfare services was rarely accompanied by any attempt to assess either effectiveness or efficiency. These two terms were largely foreign to service providers until the 1970s when pioneering and influential works such as Cochrane's (1972) study of the national health services appeared. Cochrane argued that most health care, though supposedly based on scientific principles had never been evaluated. In particular, there had been no attempt to find out whether services met their objectives (effectiveness) or whether the means of doing so were the best in terms of organization and resources (efficiency). Studies of 'outcomes' and 'value for money' ensued to meet this challenge.

With the development of major fiscal crises in western economies the need for evaluation has become ever more pressing, and, of course, more political, as cost-cutting exercises may overshadow the clarification of objectives and their attainment. Nonetheless, the study of the impact of health and welfare services has proceeded steadily in recent years, and has increasingly drawn on quality-of-life measures in doing so. In part, this is because of the reasons already outlined here, especially the limits of evaluating services on professionally derived outcomes alone (Patrick 1986: 226). The significance of survival rates, for example, may be limited in any appraisal of surgical procedures, unless we also know what quality of life the person enjoys as a result.

The use of what has come to be known as QALYS (quality-of-life adjusted years), in attempts to compare and evaluate different procedures, or services, has recently been put forward as a means of informing decisions about resource allocation. In essence, the measures attempt to bring together judgements about the quality of life under particular circumstances (for example, the impact of living with residual disability following surgery) and the number of anticipated years of survival. In this context, scientific evaluation, and moral, political, and ethical considerations, become inextricably linked, especially in the case of elderly or handicapped people, who may find that services are geared towards those groups or procedures that produce better QALYS. (For a critique of QALYS research see Loomes and McKenzie 1988).

However controversial work on QALYS has become, it has, at least, served the purpose of bringing out into the open the fact that service provision inevitably involves choices, and that evaluation research involves tackling values as well as attributes, as indeed the name itself implies. Thus, quality-of-life research involves not simply a descriptive exercise of 'mapping' the circumstances and outlook of very old people, but also the possibility of tackling evaluative issues connected with increased longevity. There are two areas where this is of particular importance for us: first, that of residential care, or what we have termed 'communal establishments', and secondly, that concerning the role of the 'informal' carers.

As we hope is clear by now, the overall position of residential care amongst the elderly must be re-examined in the case of very old people, especially amongst those aged 90 and over. Whilst it is often said that only a small proportion of the elderly live in communal establishments, our own research shows that about half of those aged 90 and over do so. Thus, concerns about the quality of life in communal establishments, loom larger in our discussion than they do in much of the general research on the elderly as a whole.

Research in this area is now growing, and involves evaluation and 'quality control' of both hospital care (Evans 1983) and other forms of public and private nursing homes and 'old people's homes' (Booth 1985; Day and Klein 1987). This in turn is feeding into the growing recognition of the need for regulation and the issuing of licences to operate communal establishments, by relevant inspectorates. This is especially important in the light of a major run-down in public provision and a rapid expansion of the private sector (Johnson 1984). Quality-of-life research among the elderly, and especially the 'oldest old', should be seen in this rapidly changing context of policy.

For example, Knapp's (1977) study of activity and life satisfaction among fifty-one residents in a southern England 'old people's home' underlined the need for communal establishments to promote active life wherever possible. The study showed that 'felt life satisfaction' was closely related to level of activity; the more active the individual was, the higher the level of life satisfaction. The reason for this may be that activity helps overcome the 'rolelessness' that old age can entail (Riley *et al.* 1988: 280); a problem that may be as important as the traditional emphasis on such matters as privacy within communal establishments, and which was recognized in the Wagner Report (1988).

The problem arises in drawing out the causal connections between variables in this kind of study – here between activity and life satisfaction. Many factors might influence the occurrence of these in residential care and, without knowing more about them, interpretations of the relationship between the two remain inconclusive. Nonetheless, research which can link levels of life satisfaction and specific areas of residential provision will gain added importance with the growth of such provision, especially in the private sector. In particular, it may help to highlight ways in which activity and autonomy may be maintained, against the tendency toward uniformity and control that communal establishments often seem to promote (Booth 1985).

Similarly, it is important in the case of very old people to focus on the role of carers in considering quality-of-life issues. The influence of relationships with family and friends (both past and present) can play a critical part in determining the quality of life, especially its emotional components. With the passing of the years, friends may die or become more distant, and relationships with family alter significantly. The problems of maintaining reciprocity or dealing with growing dependency, as well as dealing with formal carers, all raise new problems that are likely to influence the quality of life. Thus, evaluating care for the elderly increasingly involves the exploration of the dynamic interplay of formal and informal care.

Equally important is the position facing carers themselves. (Recent national evidence from the General Household Survey (GHS) has begun to document the impact of caring, especially on informal carers, mainly relatives (OPCS 1989).) Whilst it is something of a ritual today to raise the question of 'who cares for the carers?' the impact of caring for an elderly relative, and especially for one coming to the end of their life, is considerable (see e.g. Cartwright *et al.* 1973; Jones and Vetter 1984).

Two main aspects of caring have emerged from recent research, which we shall comment on further in Chapter 8 in relation to our own findings. The first of these concerns the impact of caring on the quality of life, including the health of carers themselves. The 'unremitting burden of care' (Anderson 1987) has been emphasized in a number of commentaries on the personal 'caring' aspects of community care (Bulmer 1987). It has been estimated that in 1985 there were no less than six million carers in Britain (CSO 1989a: 134), and that one household in five contained a carer. Land (in press) has pointed out that these data show that nearly one in four of these carers spend at least twenty hours a week caring, and that amongst this group a quarter of those aged between 30 and 44 years of age had a limiting long-standing illness themselves. A fifth reported that their own health had not been good in the past year. The proportions for older carers were even higher.

The second aspect of caring which has received much comment has been the sex difference in caring. A mixture of demographic factors, including of course higher death rates amongst older men, and social factors concerning roles and expectations surrounding care, has been held responsible for placing a disproportionate burden of care on female family members, especially daughters (Land 1978; Finch and Groves 1983; Ungerson 1987). Thus, it appears that men are less available to provide care, and that their expectations and abilities to care for their female partners are less than those of women. Moreover, it is often assumed that men are less able to look after themselves compared with women.

However, whilst this general picture may be true, there is a danger that the position of male carers might be overlooked. Arber and Gilbert (1989) cite several studies which have shown that between a quarter and a fifth of carers are men. Their own analysis of data from the 1980 GHS (ibid.: 116) indicates that when levels of disability are taken into account 'the major source of variation in the amount of support services received by elderly infirm men and women seems not to be the gender of the recipients or the gender of the carer but the kind of household in which they live'. This critically revolves round the availability of others to help in the informal provision of care. These aspects of caring are increasingly a feature of any evaluation of community-care policies.

Before moving on to our findings in these areas we bring into focus research that has addressed subjective quality of life for the individual in terms of experiences and events that have occurred throughout the life course. This brings together aspects of both the objective circumstances and interpersonal relationships that we have discussed so far.

SUBJECTIVE MEASURES OF THE QUALITY OF LIFE

Following our earlier delineation of quality-of-life measures, we may usefully distinguish two broad subjective dimensions here. The first concerns overall or specific kinds of 'life satisfaction' and the second concerns factors related to 'self-esteem'. Attention to the quality of life in these senses fits in well with an emphasis on biography or life course. It unlocks an investigation into the relationships between memories and perceptions people hold of the past as well as of the present and future.

A survey of the circumstances of a *current* group of very old people tells us little in itself about the 'historical' influences that have shaped the present. However, the often repeated call for longitudinal studies (e.g. Kalache *et al.* 1988) may underestimate the possibilities of studying components of the quality of life across the life course, in cross-sectional data. As Medley (1980) argues, we cannot wait fifty years to address matters of substance in the ageing field.

Relying on recall, as we have seen, has, of course, many problems, but research has been able to demonstrate some important connections between judgements of quality of life in the present, the past and the future outlook. Staats and Stasson (1987), for example, show that future expectations of the quality of life are closely linked to current outlook in that present happiness or unhappiness colours perceptions of the future. Stones and Kozma (1986) put this in the context of 'propensities' built up over time. By this they mean that the outlook of elderly people, as it has developed through significant phases of the life course, creates a 'cognitive style' which informs decision-making in day-to-day settings. This, in turn, creates a 'propensity' for the situation to become self-fulfilling in the future, though of course this is not an ineluctable causal sequence. Over time people seek out those circumstances where their underlying philosophy of life is reinforced. This philosophy of life, and its formation in historically specific circumstances, provides a sense of continuity between personal and public events.

At the personal level, the term 'events' refers here to two sets of experiences. The first are the anticipated events that structure the life course of most individuals (which we alluded to in our 'life tree' in Chapter 3, p.45); leaving the parental home, setting up a home of one's own, marriage and children, the breaking away of children, exiting from the labour market and possible bereavement in later life. The full range of these events is, of course, particularly relevant to the very long lived.

The second are those events that cut across hopes and expectations; the loss of a child, or of a job, the onset of poor health or the unexpected experience of bereavement (in our study, for example, an instance of the loss of a son in a plane crash). Much of the research on 'life events' concentrates, in adult life, on this latter group of events and their impact on mental health, especially through their lowering of self-esteem (see e.g. Brown and Harris 1978; Andrews and Brown 1988). Here, we wish to comment briefly on the role of both sorts of events in terms of life satisfaction as well as self-esteem.

Research on the experience of events across a long life course reveals how important their timing is. It seems clear that most of us operate with a definite 'social clock' which guides our expectations of events within the biographical context (for a broader discussion of time and the life course see Young 1988). Such expectations influence whether events are anticipated or unanticipated, the latter having more negative implications for the quality of life than the former. For example, to suffer the onset of a serious disabling illness at an early age, particularly in a historical setting where such an occurrence is relatively rare, can create a sense of being 'cheated' out of expected life stages (Bury 1982).

Such biographical disruption is likely to have profound effects on the response of the individual to subsequent experiences. As argued earlier, the onset of disabling illness in later life may be accompanied by a greater sense of acceptance or even stoicism. It may be that biographical timing rather than passivity helps explain such acceptance, a factor that needs to be borne in mind in proposals for more active medical treatment for the very old.

Fallo-Mitchell and Ryff (1982) draw attention to two key variations in the nature of 'social clocks' which are important for our discussion. First, they argue that different birth cohorts may have quite different expectations of events. Thus, expectations of the age at which one should marry or leave the parental home may be significantly influenced by cultural patterns as well as individual variations. The entry to and exit from age-related 'role structures' is governed by structural features and people's active response to them (Riley et al. 1988: 251). Perhaps many of the clashes between generations are to do with the 'clash of clocks' implied here.

Second, there are potentially significant differences in expectations between the sexes. Fallo-Mitchell and Ryff (1982: 265) review the expectations of women across the life cycle and conclude that their findings 'suggest the existence of social clocks that serve to sanction the appropriate times for events in the female life cycle'. Serious departures from such expected timings may have important influences on the quality of life, especially for women who may be particularly affected by such events. Overall life satisfaction continues to rise for men across the life course, even into later years, whereas it tends to 'plateau' for women (Medley 1980: 198). As we shall see, this is of particular relevance to our own study of very old people.

At a social psychological level, it has also proved useful to investigate the impact of past experiences and events on the quality of life. Murphy (1982) has provided evidence to link both personality factors and life events in the past with current mental-health status. In a study of elderly people suffering from depression, she was able to show that poor relationships prior to the onset of old age were significantly associated with the current onset of illness. Low self-esteem and unhappiness brought over from the past into old age, increased vulnerability to depression in the face of life events, such as bereavement or physical illness.

Those who had experienced good relationships in the past were more likely to be able to withstand the impact of changes and negative events in old age. As Murphy reminds us, 'T'is better to have loved and lost than never to have loved at all.' Thus, good experiences in the past can have a considerable bearing on the present. They may reduce vulnerability to the negative effects of threatening life events. Needless to say, the causal pathways between events and quality of life, are difficult to establish, and it is not the purpose of the present study to try to do so. What is clear, however, is that negative or unanticipated events do not produce serious effects on self-worth or self-esteem in any simple way. Coping mechanisms may intervene to offset the impact of events or bolster a vulnerable personality.

In this connection, research on the impact of social and leisure activities and of social support on the quality of life is of importance. The distinction between objective and subjective dimensions is difficult to sustain here, as these factors might more properly be seen as objective indicators of quality of life in their own right. Be that as it may, there is considerable evidence that patterns of social life, including leisure activities, influence the quality of life.

Remaining active and having adequate social support are likely to contribute to the quality of life in a residential setting. As Bulmer (1987: 60), however, has recently argued, patterns of social ties and activities vary considerably in adult life, and these may have lasting effects on expectations. He points out that in adult life, middle-class or professional groups have extensive social networks often based on work during adult life, compared with working-class groups who do not (for a more general discussion of these class differences, see Allan 1979). This kind of variation warns against making too many assumptions about the role of social activities and support across the life course.

Mutran and Reitzes (1981) provide a useful approach to the linking of activities with both broader social indicators and objective measures on the one hand, and with well-being on the other.

In this way it is possible to address more 'mediated' links that might help predict well-being. Among very old people, as we shall see, many activities may be noticeable by being either severely reduced or absent, though this is not always the case. By the age of 90, well-being may be predicated on a more 'passive' life style in the present, though, of course, valued memories of social life in the past may remain intact. Moreover, in very old age it may be that satisfaction with leisure is more important than activity itself (Ragheb and Griffiths 1982).

In summary, subjective measures of the quality of life, such as those of life satisfaction, well-being or self-esteem, direct our attention to important events and their effects on individuals throughout the life course. They also relate to important changes in the position of the very old in a changing social environment. Our own emphasis on the subjective dimensions of very old age means that we should give considerable weight to the interaction between these components. We take this further in the ensuing three chapters.

6

EVERYDAY LIFE

We now turn to some of those subjective measures and evaluations of the quality of life, discussed in the previous chapter. We look at what daily life is like for very old people and the extent to which such feelings as boredom, loneliness and worry are experienced. We also see whether they look forward to the day, what things, such as religious beliefs, family and friends, give pleasure or support, and how very old people themselves regard old age. All these aspects of their lives and feelings are examined in the round, taking note of their possible association with the elderly individuals' health and disability and their socio-economic circumstances. Differences arising from life in a domiciliary or a communal setting are noted.

PASSING THE TIME

All through life, from infancy to extreme old age, how people pass the time is largely a matter of habit dictated by individual propensities and circumstances, tempered by the customs and condition of society, past and present. The broad sweep of change intrinsic to the life course is obvious, combining both 'cyclical' and 'linear' elements in the passage of time (Young 1988).

Even in the first years of life there are marked differences in everyday activities according to culture, parental circumstances and beliefs, the child's health and responses. By the age of 90, a great divergence could be expected, dependent on the accumulation, and influences, of earlier differences in circumstances on individual capacities and temperament. At the same time, reaching extreme old age, which inevitably entails the partial shedding or the loss of many of the consequences of those influences, might in itself bring about more homogeneity. How far, then, would the differences and similarities already apparent in the various aspects of their lives we have so far considered also appear in the way very old people pass the time? One way to discover this was to ask them to describe a typical day.

A typical day

To expect from the elderly people a uniformly full account of their typical day was clearly unrealistic. Memory was sometimes poor; there was considerable variation in the content of the days. Many were uneventful. Sometimes an account could be short but representative of a full life, or the opposite, though an uneventful day need not mean that the quality of that person's life is correspondingly poor. Similar daily routines were not always regarded in the same way.

Mrs Salter, for example, aged 95 and the widow of a policeman, spoke contentedly of her seemingly routine existence. Living in a local authority home for the past four years, she told the interviewer she was happy there. She had worked in a fruit shop from the age of 13 until her marriage and had lived all her life in the same town. Her memory was poor – the past 'just went on ordinary' – and now she needed help with dressing, toileting and bathing. She never felt lonely and got on well with her fellow residents. Her typical day was as follows:

> I wake up at seven a.m. and have a glass of orange juice. I wash my face and hands in my room. I get dressed with some help and have my hair combed. I don't mind that, though I could do it myself. I go down for breakfast at eight o'clock – in a wheelchair. I have cornflakes. I get taken into the lounge after breakfast. I just sit and chat – the TV is on all day but I don't take much interest in it. I have a cup of milk during the morning. I have lunch and then go back in the lounge. I sometimes doze off in my chair. Tea is at five p.m. Then back to the lounge. I stay downstairs until after I've had a drink and then I get taken up to bed. I have a bath once a week.

When she has visitors – her son or grandson and their wives – she gets taken up to her room. She doesn't join in any bingo or read, nor does she go out at all.

Underlying Mrs Hopkins' day in a residential home, though described in terms similar to those of Mrs Salter, was the spectre of despair, as was discovered from her replies to later questions.

> I get up early – just after eight o'clock and they bring my

breakfast up to me. I try to get out of my room so they can clean it and I go downstairs and sit in the lounge. I watch television when there's anything on. I have a cup of tea in the afternoon and my meal at six o'clock. They bring my hot water bottle up to me at ten o'clock and I am usually in bed at eleven.

Mr Compton, the blind ex-sailor with 'rum in his veins', living with his daughter, described his day at length.

I wake up between seven and eight a.m. Don't get up until eleven or twelve o'clock! Just lie in bed and listen to the radio. I don't even bother with tea in bed. I get up for the WC and then go back to bed. I get up and wash and dress on my own. I come down for breakfast at about 12 noon. My daughter has made it.

After breakfast I listen to the radio and have a pipe, sitting in the comfortable chair in the kitchen. My daughter leaves lunch for me, which I eat at about three o'clock.

I fall asleep in the chair for an hour or so quite often during the afternoon when there's nothing interesting on the radio. I've got everything handy there. I don't go upstairs to rest but climb the stairs two to three times a day to the WC. I come down backwards – like a ship's ladder. We all have the evening meal together at between half past six to seven o'clock. My food needs cutting up. I see the grandchildren when they come in from school.

During the evening I listen to the radio with headphones. I get myself to bed without help. I do my own eyedrops.

Relatively bald statements may, as in the case of Mr Craddock, aged 91, conceal a life involving a much wider range of activities than that of Mr Compton, as corroborated by his replies to other questions and confirmed by his daughter.

Mr Craddock lived alone but walked every day to have dinner with his daughter who lived nearby. His choice of a 'typical day' was a Sunday.

I got up and had breakfast – usually toasted white bread – washed, shaved and made my bed. Then I got dressed and went to my daughter's. I always go to morning service with her at the Salvation Army. At half past ten. I had my lunch with my daughter; read the paper, went to afternoon service and then evening service. I was brought home by car at about half past eight.

Mrs Johnson described her day with enthusiasm and in considerable detail. She had been in service before her marriage and had lived in the same little end-of-terrace house for sixty years. Alone now but surrounded by devoted children and grandchildren living nearby, she gave the following account of her day:

> I wake at about eight o'clock. I think that is the time to get up. I put the wireless on and listen to the news. I have a cup of tea. I get my breakfast – I go in for plain living – bread and butter and marmalade; I don't cook breakfast.
>
> During the morning I do the fireside [a coal fire], dusting and then do the bedrooms. My daughter comes in for a 'bit of a chat'. I get on with my work – the bedrooms. I have a washing machine but mainly do the washing by hand. My daughter has an automatic so she does the sheets.
>
> I have dinner – a proper one: meat, veg, potatoes, soup. Then do the washing up. In the afternoon I have a nap on the settee in the sitting room for just half an hour. I watch the TV if there's anything on. I maybe write a letter to my son – my granddaughter copies it out. The family visits. I make my own tea – a sandwich or an egg, salad, cakes. I still do my own baking, but I have difficulty measuring out the ingredients because of my eyesight! I make scones once a week.
>
> During the evening I watch TV. My daughter calls. My grandson calls occasionally and my granddaughter calls every evening. A neighbour sometimes calls for a chat. I have a cup of tea and go to bed at ten o'clock.

These few 'typical days', and other accounts of daily life given earlier and later in this book, are not easy to interpret. Descriptions of the routine nature of the daily round can both illuminate and disguise the quality of life. Some individuals described a range of activities providing evidence of a good quality of life, whilst 'inactivity' could bring feelings of satisfaction or dissatisfaction to others.

Prescriptions for a happy old age are often contradictory, emphasizing both the need to remain active and the need to 'take things easy'. Moreover, both activities and feelings are partly determined by where and with whom the individuals live. Mrs Johnson, for instance, seemed glad to fill a large part of the day spent on her own with household

Table 6.1 Frequency of indoor leisure activities: weighted sample

Activities	Often %	Sometimes %	Never %	Total no. of subjects = 171–179 %
Chatting, talking	47.5	36.7	15.8	100
Watching TV	43.6	29.1	27.4	100[1]
Reading	40.4	8.4	51.1	100[1]
Watching people go by	56.1	17.0	26.9	100
Listening to radio	26.3	30.7	43.0	100
Playing cards, etc.	6.1	7.3	86.6	100
Other crafts	4.6	4.0	91.4	100
Other, including listening to and making music, gardening	24.8	11.7	63.4	100[1](145)

[1]See note 2.

chores. But, as we have seen, the typical day does not only involve household routines and chores; other pursuits need to be brought into the picture to help in the interpretive task.

'Leisure' activities

We have enclosed the word leisure in quotes because the day for nonagenarians and centenarians cannot really be divided into work and leisure periods. But it serves to distinguish what we shall now be discussing from the activities of daily living (ADLs) discussed in Chapter 4. Table 6.1 shows how often indoor leisure activities occurred.

Just under half the total sample 'often' watched television, and here it was noticeable that among members of the actual sample proportionately fewer of the older age groups did so. Over one-quarter of the sample never watched television and under one-third sometimes did. It is reported that the population aged 65 and over as a whole watch an average of nearly thirty-seven and a half hours of television a week (CSO 1989(a): table 10.4). When we compare this with our findings, it appears that people aged 90 and over watch relatively little. The proportions of people with poor eyesight or severe confusion partly account for this, though it might also have something to do with the fact that, as a generation, television entered their lives after leisure habits were formed. This might suggest that listening to the radio would be more popular, in terms of regular or frequent listening, than watching television but here, as was confirmed by a cross-check, the high prevalence of deafness was certainly instrumental in relegating it to fifth place in the order of popularity.

Reading books and newspapers was mentioned by just under half the sample, the great majority of these reading 'often'. Given the problem of eyesight, this suggests that, for those able to, reading remains an important activity in very old people's lives. Mr Crawford, for instance, settled daily in the public library before eleven o'clock. He was, at the time of the interview, reading Bertrand Russell's *Why I am not a Christian*; he had 'given up fiction'. Mr Morgan played the piano every day – 'Music has always been very important to me. I still play records', as did a handful of others. Watching people go by was clearly much appreciated, something of which elderly residents on upper floors or surrounded by gardens often feel much deprived.

Only relatively small proportions of the sample used their hands in leisure pursuits, though DIY occurred as an activity in one or two instances, and knitting was mentioned by a quarter of the younger women and one man. Mrs Johnson was not alone in still being able to sew, despite a problem she had in threading needles. This was overcome by getting them threaded for her, several at a time, and stuck in the curtain. Mrs Warner was making cushion covers 'at the moment' and also knitted. Puzzles kept others amused, a bit of gardening was managed by a few.

Games and chat need other people. Mrs Johnson bemoaned the fact that there was 'no-one left to play cards with' though Mrs Stratton, aged 96, living in a private residential home, undaunted by her blindness, in constant pain but with high morale, 'paid someone to play bingo' for her.

But talking and chatting was most popular of all, engaged in, (either often or sometimes), by the great majority of the total sample. The opportunities for chat and talk would, it might be thought, be greater in a communal than in a domiciliary setting, especially if in the latter they were living alone. In fact, this last group were proportionately amongst the largest who mentioned it, topping those living communally by nearly 20 per cent. Otherwise, people living in residential homes, and sometimes nursing homes, were, on the whole, as likely to engage in many of the specified leisure activities as those living in private households. This was particularly true for radio listening, reading, needlework or knitting. Noticeably fewer people, however, living in residential or nursing homes watched TV often. Thus, on another level, a distinction between the frequency with which leisure activities that rely only on the individual for their execution and those dependent on other people seems not to depend on the immediate availability of others. There was little difference between men and women in the extent of their indoor leisure activities.

In considering outdoor activities we have to remember that we are talking about a markedly smaller group – the non-housebound – than the total sample. Men, as we know, went out of doors significantly more often than women. Beyond this, however, much depends on what they do when they go out. We have earlier distinguished between the occasional, accompanied stroll down the road and the regular unaccompanied walk (see Chapter 4). Mr Craddock belonged to the latter group. His daughter elaborated the ritual of his daily walk:

> He doesn't come the short way – he comes the furthest way round and the same going home. If it's raining too heavily he will go straight home but on the other hand, if it's raining just ordinary and he's got his raincoat and umbrella, he will still go the long way round. It's no good telling him not to do it. He says, 'If I were to give up I would just sit and do nothing and go nowhere but while I can do it I will.'

Being taken for a drive – usually by a member of the family – was enjoyed by just under half the total non-housebound sample, and shopping expeditions – sometimes alone but more often accompanied – by one-third. 'My daughter's been a darling to me', Mrs Arthur told the interviewer. 'We go out when she comes and usually buy some new clothes.' But the outdoor activity undertaken by the largest proportion of the sample (three-quarters) was visits to family and friends, either alone or accompanied.

As with indoor leisure activities so with outdoor – the private household/communal divide was not uniform or predictable, though the different sizes of the groups demand caution in making comparisons; there were nearly twice as many replying to the question in the private household group. With this in mind, we found, excluding hospital patients, that something under two-fifths of those living in residential, or even nursing, homes went for walks, either alone or accompanied, compared with roughly similar proportions of those living with others in private households. It was those living alone – over two-fifths – who formed the largest group. Not very dissimilar proportions living in the two main settings went to see family or friends, either alone or accompanied. This suggests that, although relatively fewer people in the communal setting go out-of-doors, entry into an establishment does not necessarily entail the relinquishment of outdoor pursuits.

Going to the shops, as would be expected, was more likely to occur among the non-communal group than among their counterparts, but only by a small margin. With club attendance, on the other hand, there was virtually no difference between the two groups – just over one-third of those living alone or with others, and the same for those in residential homes.

Returning to the quantity of leisure activity reported, Mrs Arthur and Mrs Warner specified the highest number of indoor activities engaged in, seven in all, and both went out of doors. Here is Mrs Arthur, who, somewhat unusually for someone in a residential home, had a low level of disability.

> I watch tennis on the TV – I'm a tennis fiend. Then there's knitting – I'm knitting vests for Mother Theresa's babies. I read big-print books. I do crosswords and play scrabble. I used to give talks up to last November [she is a Women's Guild member] and I still get thoughts in my mind. I think I shall be preparing another talk. Every Wednesday I walk to the church for a coffee and a chat. I crochet my handkerchiefs, I never use tissues. I love my tapestry. I've been mending pillowslips today. I have been a patron of the Little Theatre for years and years and years but I won't be going there this year because the steps are too difficult. I write all my prayers down.

Mrs Warner, as well as sewing and knitting regularly, played bingo once a week. 'I never played bingo until I came here [to a sheltered housing unit] and now I'm a dab hand at it. I go to Red Cross meetings on Mondays and I play whist. I do watch TV but prefer the wireless.'

But, as we have indicated, being 'busy' or filling one's days does not necessarily require a great variety of activity. The only leisure activities mentioned by Mr Ross, for instance, were watching TV occasionally and playing cards often, yet he was himself convinced of the importance of being busy. One of the car drivers, a 93-year-old ex-naval widower, he lived independently in a sheltered housing flat with a 'house mother' on call, if necessary. For him the time went 'too quickly':

> I have so much to do – am fully occupied. In a place like this there

is only one to do the dinners the same as if there was two or three and they can share it. And then there's making the bed, changing the sheets, getting the laundry ready – it all takes time.

Mrs Forbes was another without a long list of activities to her name, yet, according to the deputy matron of her rest home, she kept her mind fully occupied. 'She reads the paper every day and lots of library books, and she writes masses of letters.'

As we suggested in Chapter 5, and have already seen in the various illustrations, the relationship between activity and quality of life, if the latter is assessed by levels of subjective contentment, is a tenuous one. Mr Brandon exemplifies the mix of objective circumstances and subjective evaluations. He lived in a local authority home and was unable to do anything for himself except feeding. From this point of view, his quality of life might be categorized as poor. He was blind, had a cleft palate and hare lip, was generally exceedingly frail and said he was in pain. Yet he told the interviewer that he usually looked forward to the day and when asked if he was happy where he was, he said: 'Yes, I'd be happy anywhere.' It appeared that he lived largely in the past and fantasized about the present. When asked why he thought he had lived so long, he replied, 'I think I have an innocent mind.'

MORALE

This area of questioning proved more difficult than those relying on a factual basis, and resulted in fewer replies. This is mainly because proxies, by definition, could not draw on subjective views. The topics under our heading of 'morale', nevertheless, provide a further guide to subjective well-being among the very old.

Boredom

We, like others, asked the sample members if they had any difficulty in passing the time. Of those replying to the question, the majority, something over three-fifths, said that they had no difficulty (see Table 6.2).

Nearly twice as many women as men said that they were bored, though feelings were not always consistent. Mrs Forbes, for instance, despite her busy life, and the comments of the deputy matron reported above, sometimes found the days go quickly and 'sometimes', she said,

they drag a little. I miss not being able to do any odd jobs such as

Table 6.2 Self-perceptions of boredom: weighted sample

Experienced	%
No	62.8
Yes	37.2
Total subjects	100
	(140)

putting on a button – I can't see to thread a needle. But I have got accustomed to it – not being able to do the things I used to.

This comparison with the past was asked for in our questioning. Just over half the total sample of those replying said they found it more difficult to pass the time now than in earlier times. Like Mrs Forbes, they mainly gave as their reason that they were no longer able to do what they used to do. Of those claiming that their feelings in this respect were unchanged, some took a positive line, referring to their 'attitude of mind' or 'active brain' and the support they gave to family and friends, while others spoke of resignation, 'taking things as they come' and so on.

We naturally looked to see if there was an association between boredom, or the lack of it, and some of the other factors we have considered in this and previous chapters. In the total sample, as might be expected, restrictions on mobility were associated with a higher level of boredom. When, however, we look at the experiences of particular groups, these do not always fit the general pattern. Over three-quarters, for example, of the housebound group managing without aid said they had no difficulty in passing the time, compared with just under two-thirds of those who could go out on their own. Thus, for Mr Compton, housebound and blind, the time passed 'pretty well. I don't get tired of life.' And in answer to why he thought this was, he replied, 'Just a contented mind, that's all.'

Here we have a hint of the attraction of considering attitudes in relation to the life course, not so much in terms of circumstances as of temperament and intellectual resources. Mr Compton's 'contented mind' was not, we suspect from the account of his life and his daughter's comments, anything new. People do, of course, change. It is a cliché that mellowing comes with age, though it has been said that 'a tart temper never mellows'. Moreover, though there was a significant association between lack of boredom and the activities of reading or needlework and knitting, if someone has in the past had many interests, inability to indulge them now because of physical or mental impairment may not be so disastrous, since they may yet provide in retrospect a source of strength and contentment. Thus, inability to carry out activities does not necessarily impair self-esteem.

The presence of others was significant in alleviating boredom. Over half those living alone, for example, said they had difficulty in passing the time compared with well under one-third of those in private households, and just over one-quarter of those living in residential or nursing homes. Mrs James, for instance, the youngest of nine children and the widow of a groom, with an above-average level of disability, a sense of humour and 'much loved', it seems, by the staff of her nursing home, was 'never bored'. She knitted, read novels, and helped others whenever she could, including, it may be remembered, lending her hearing aid. She was 'looking after' a centenarian fellow resident at the time of the interview.

But, as we have already seen, some of those living alone also succeeded in filling their time effectively. Mr Anderson, with a very low level of disability, who lived next door to his daughter – 'if I want anything I knock on the wall and she comes round' – was never bored. He had a young dog that he was still training and said he would take her out every day to exercise her when she was a little older. He liked gardening and doing DIY jobs around the house.

The diversity in the pattern of responses about boredom, confirms our earlier contention that, for most, the propensity for boredom has origins and remedies which do not necessarily depend on what you do or cannot do. Is the same true of loneliness, another important indicator of well-being?

Loneliness

By considering the question of loneliness through subjective evaluation, we do at least avoid the pitfall of attempting to define it 'through the eye of the beholder' (Brearley 1982: 42). This, however, does not make it much easier to explain; as elsewhere in a consideration of the quality of life, there are always the hazards of interpretation. A strong association, nevertheless, exists in old age between loneliness and bereavement, particularly 'the emotional trauma caused by the loss of a life companion' (Age Concern 1974: 44-5). Perhaps, as can be seen in Table 6.3, one reason for the relatively small proportion – fewer than one-fifth – of the sample who said that they often experienced

Table 6.3 Self-perceptions of loneliness: weighted sample

Experienced	%
Never	60.5
Sometimes	32.2
Often	7.3
Total subjects	100
	(148)

loneliness was the fact that for many, the major bereavement of their spouse had occurred some considerable time before they were interviewed.

The exceptions were poignantly exemplified by Mrs Ricketts who said she felt 'ready for the rubbish tip'. She was still, it seems, grieving for the husband she had lost twenty years before and her two sons, killed in air crashes. Her daughter-in-law and grandchildren lived in Canada and 'neglected' her. Mrs Trench, who exceptionally had lost her husband only the previous week, was, according to the interviewer and not surprisingly, in a low state.

So in these two examples, as we discussed in Chapter 5, we have an instance of the meeting point between objective circumstances (bereavement) and meaning for the individual (loneliness and sadness). There is, furthermore, a 'conceptual distinction between isolation and loneliness' (Tinker 1984: 163). 'Isolation relates to *circumstances* (which can usually be measured, however crudely), whereas loneliness relates to feelings (often about those circumstances)' (ibid).

Our findings generally on perceived loneliness and frequency of social contact agree in the main with those of other studies of elderly people (see e.g. Shanas *et al.* 1968: 271; Victor 1987: 235-6; Bowling *et al.* 1988: 23). The evidence suggests that lack of social contact does not necessarily engender a sense of loneliness. 'Social contact', however, is in our view an inadequate measure since, though 'frequent' it may be fleeting, and vice versa. Although we found (on the basis of small numbers) relatively little difference between the feelings of those in frequent and infrequent contact with relatives and friends, where they were living with relatives, over three-quarters said they never felt lonely. This suggests that 'company' rather than contact means more to the very old.

This was borne out by the fact that there was a significant

association between feelings of loneliness and the number of hours a day spent alone. Again, this broad grouping subsumes many variations. Over three-quarters of those living in private households who always had company, never felt lonely, and none reported that they 'often' did. Conversely, of the group who spent from twelve to twenty-four hours a day on their own, nearly two-thirds said that they felt lonely sometimes or often. Mrs Benson, isolated by extreme deafness and unable to stand without a frame, belonged to this group, though her meals were provided by her niece (except for meals-on-wheels on Mondays) and she had a weekly 'washdown' by a nurse and paid a weekly visit to hospital by ambulance; her husband had died fifty years before. Her reply to the question was, 'Lonely? That's what I am, I am lonely. When I'm sitting here I am ever so pleased when I hear that door because it means someone is coming.' Women in the sample voiced feelings of loneliness proportionately more often than men.

There is a marginal difference between the feelings of those living in a communal setting compared with those in a domestic one – the former experiencing loneliness less often than the latter. But, even in a communal environment, as Mr Charles testified, special companionship is important in counteracting loneliness. It was, he said,

worse now, because when we had the bad weather at the beginning of the year my two friends had accidents and had to go into hospital. Also I was always used to being busy and now, when things have all eased up, my companions have gradually gone.

The general spirits of members of the sample, as we saw in Chapter 4, were good and, with some qualification, we have found that general morale was also often good. But such assessments of general well-being need to be set against specific areas of worry.

Worries

People may be strongly motivated to respond to questions about mood in positive terms – admitting loneliness and boredom may not be acceptable. Moreover, how well people are coping with the demands of everyday life in general says little about what aspects of life are most troublesome. With this in mind, we asked about a range of possible concerns. Promptings covered such possible worries as their own health, the health of others close to them, money, their living arrangements, the fear of being a burden, the idea of death. Under each of these headings the majority said they did not worry, though responses varied. Mrs Dodds, unusually for members of this sample, worried about her 'memory loss'. The most notable worry was concern for others, either in the shape of their health or their caring role. Mrs Horden, for example, worried over her family 'if they're not well'. One of her sons had had 'a lot of bad luck and sickness'.

Worries about being a burden were expressed by just under one-quarter of the elderly individuals replying to the question. Mrs Hopkins, when asked if she went out for a walk, replied, 'I'm always terrified I'll be a nuisance to anybody, so I don't ask.' Mr Abbott, when asked about worries said, 'I always say I am just a damn nuisance and I am.' A few were by their own admission just worriers – Mr Robinson said he was 'the biggest worrier on earth. I worry about anything, but never myself. I worry over any little thing.'

The concern about being a burden may, both in its origins in everyday experience and the social expectations surrounding very old age, be a reflection of 'structured dependency', resulting from social attitudes towards old age rather than the 'objective' needs of the individual, and creating a complicated picture which it is difficult to disentangle. What is clear, however, is that both the present fact of being cared for or its likely imminence, and the expectation that this will be a burden for someone, may exert a negative influence on well-being.

Regardless of worries, most people on waking, if not seriously depressed, are able to accommodate themselves to the day ahead. Whether or not they look forward to each day is another matter.

Looking forward to the day

The nonagenarians and centenarians of our sample at the time of their interview were waking up and contemplating the day ahead for something in the region of the thirty-five thousandth time in their lives. This fact gives a sense of perspective to the years and days which have hitherto constituted their life course. It would not in our view have been surprising to find many for whom another day was just one too many, who might say, with Mrs Hopkins, 'My God, not another blinking, empty day.' But not so; as can be seen from Table 6.4, only a small minority, when asked whether they looked forward to the day on waking, replied in negative terms ('never' or 'rarely'), and as many as 65 per cent replied 'usually'.

We then looked to see what might account for those differences in

Table 6.4 Looking forward to the day on waking: weighted sample

	%
Usually	65.1
Sometimes	6.6
Indifferent	17.6
Rarely	5.5
Never	5.2
Total subjects	100
	(142)

outlook. The minorities suffering constant pain, for instance, or serious problems of incontinence, might correspond with the minority who never or rarely looked forward to the day. Conversely, we might expect to find that those able to go out would be more inclined to take a positive view of the day ahead than those who could not. There were indeed some significant associations, but, as we by now were prepared to find, the patterns were not consistent. Even where they were, the causal direction of such associations is open to doubt.

The degree of mobility did appear to have some association with their feelings in the matter. Nearly three times as many of the housebound, compared with those going out, for example, rarely or never looked forward to the day.Not going for drives seems to have dampened their pleasurable anticipation somewhat more than inability to go shopping or to church or to a club. It is possible, however, that mobility is itself affected by morale; those with low morale are less likely to be motivated to go out.

Incontinence, of either kind, seems to have made no difference to looking forward to the day, which is surprising, and pain, only marginally. The worst sufferers were more-or-less equally divided in their views. Mrs Nisbett, for instance, aged 96, despite a constant pain from shingles 'just below the shoulder', usually looked forward to the day. She lived with her daughter and son-in-law, enjoyed the radio, television, needlework, cards and chat, but was 'more fond of reading than anything else'; reading, it may be remembered, functioned as her 'sleeping pill'. Mrs Holland, by contrast, never looked forward to the day and was 'just sitting waiting to die'. Partial confusion (her daughter, with whom she lived, part-proxied the interview) and the pain caused by severe arthritis allowed her only to listen to the radio and occasionally chat.

Mr Abbott was another who never looked forward to the day. His situation exemplified that mix of circumstance and temperament which together may influence feelings. Circumstances, of course, include 'others', and in this particular case there had, it seems, been a recent altercation with the matron of his home. From the interview it is not clear what role the matron may have played in this except that she had, it appears, vetoed an attempt by Mr Abbott to arrange his own lift to the barber's.

Those of the sample living alone appeared to be less inclined to look forward to the day – 38 per cent replying 'never', 'rarely' or 'indifferent' compared with 14 per cent of those living with others and 31 per cent of those replying resident in all types of communal establishment.

Although these are all minorities, they nevertheless comprise a substantial proportion of people for whom, in anticipation at least, the day held little or nothing pleasurable. Even contact with relatives failed to stimulate an interest.

There is, however, no doubt that, in general, close family ties act as a buffer between circumstances and low self-esteem. The importance for very old people of personal relationships – mainly with the family – came to light especially in replies to a question on what gave pleasure and support.

What gave pleasure and support?

Of those replying to this question, 40 per cent talked either exclusively or mostly of personal relationships. Otherwise they mainly mentioned the various activities which we have already discussed. Pleasures to do with the senses such as food, 'a smoke', 'a Guiness', were mentioned by a few. Mr Proctor, aged 102, when asked the question, just showed his pipe with a gold lid to the bowl – 'the waggoner I used to plough for said "I will give you a pipe if you want to smoke" and I've had it ever since' – and his 'baccy box', a beautiful silver box containing his block tobacco. He added, 'I like a humbug now and again.' Pets were mentioned by only a handful. Quite a substantial minority – two-fifths – said that they got pleasure from their surroundings – 'the sunshine', 'watching the birds' or their garden. A smaller, very positive, group did not bother to discriminate, replying 'everything' or 'almost everything'.

It is clear that personal relationships not only gave pleasure but also support, and this we shall be discussing more fully in the next chapters.

There was, however, a small minority who made little of them generally. Perhaps they had always been 'loners'; one or two said as much.

Another element in the lives of very old people that we assumed might be important was religious faith. Church-going has declined steadily in recent years, but in the time of their youth and early middle age it would have been more common among those now in their 90s and beyond. In the latter half of the nineteenth century some 40 per cent of the British population attended church, whilst today only 10 per cent do so (Abercrombie et al 1988: 434).

Of the group replying to a question about their religious beliefs, 57 per cent averred that these did give them support. Mr Godwin told the interviewer that he could

> talk to Jesus – he's my greatest friend today. God would always look after me; if I am worried I can ask for certain things. One thing that gives me great confidence for the future is 'Songs of Praise' – people with enthusiasm, and the children; it makes a tremendous difference.

The popularity of the BBC television programme 'Songs of Praise' appears to be widespread among older people. Though younger, more secularized, generations may react to such programmes with amusement, the idea of television as a form of reassurance (Taylor and Mullen 1986) gains some credibility here. For those unable to go out, or attend church in person, television programmes like 'Songs of Praise' offer an important substitute, and source of pleasure.

For Mrs Arthur, religion had been 'the most important thing' in her life. 'If I hadn't had faith when my husband died I couldn't have carried on.' Mr Alcock, living alone in a sheltered housing unit, turned his strong religious beliefs to the advantage of others, by 'offering' himself 'in the event of anyone in the unit wanting any spiritual help' [he had hoped to go into the Ministry].

There was a small minority who felt uncertainty, who 'would like to believe', felt that it was all 'a mystery', but who did not seem to be perturbed at their lack of positive faith. Others again, in roughly similar proportions, were positive in their non-belief – they were not 'interested', thought it all 'fiction or fantasy', or even 'rubbish'. This had always been so with them, or they had lost their one-time belief, seemingly without regret. And then there were the 'philosophers' – two or three and male – of whom Mr Unwin is a fair example: 'I believe all religions are all codes of ethics. We don't know anything about God. I have come to think about death as a blessed relief from the burden of existence.'

Feelings about place of residence

The state of an individual's morale is almost bound to be influenced by his or her feelings about where she or he lives. It is important, therefore, that, irrespective of whether they were living privately or communally, the majority of the elderly people in our study said they had no wish to move. Altogether, out of 150 members of the actual sample replying to the question, only eleven women and nine men, of whom seven and four respectively were in private households, said they would like to move.

In private households, sample members spoke of being 'settled', 'happy' or 'contented'; they were near their families or had good neighbours. A few felt they were 'too old to move', were reluctant to give up their own home or their independence, or had 'nowhere better to go'.

The kinds of reasons generally offered by those in communal establishments for wishing to stay were similar to those of the private household group, though more emphasis was given to the quality of the care they received. There were more, perhaps, in this group than among those in private households who, in saying they wished to move, recognized at the same time that the idea was unrealistic. Mr Fletcher, for example, who lived in a local authority home with his wife, was himself fit and active though blind, enjoying the radio, records and chat. He longed to move out to a home of their own but his wife needed the nursing care provided by the home and which he was unable to give.

Mrs Plater, aged 98, doubly incontinent and very frail, was another with unrealistic, if understandable, desires. She was in a private residential home whither she had gone four years previously after numerous falls. She said she was 'happy here in a way', and the home was very suitable in the interviewer's opinion. But 'There's no place like home. I'd go home tomorrow if I could.'

For the communal sample, to try to get nearer to the realities of daily life in a single interview, we followed up these questions about moving or staying with ones concerning their living arrangements. First, in general terms, the message coming through the replies was one of satisfaction, over half replying 'definitely' satisfied, and just under two-fifths 'on the whole'.

As a further check we singled out twelve particular items for them to consider. The numbers replying were relatively small, about half the establishment-based sample. Nevertheless, among these, with some exceptions, there was a high level of satisfaction concerning both the types of establishment and particular arrangements. About cupboard and drawer space, for instance, despite the relatively poor provision in council homes, or about sleeping arrangements, there was very little complaint. Mr Proctor showed the interviewer a big chest in his room, filled with his grandfather's and his own tools. Mrs Jessop was unhappy at having to share a room and Miss Flint, though generally content, did not like her room. This was mainly a matter of privacy – 'People try to get in when I'm not there.' The shrinkage of owned 'territory' from a whole home to one room may understandably generate suspicions which are in truth unfounded. Lack of privacy as such, however, was complained of by only four people.

Otherwise there were individual criticisms of the facilities for bathing and washing, for personal belongings, sleeping arrangements, the food and recreational facilities. On this last point, while some homes certainly did seem to offer opportunities for recreation, including outings, no innovative schemes were evident, and in many homes there appeared to be nothing other than the inevitable television.

The few adverse comments were spread across the different types of establishment – local authority, voluntary and private. No one sample member voiced more than two or three criticisms. In the very few establishments housing more than one sample member, they were not criticized for the same failings by more than one resident. The area giving rise to the most expressions of dissatisfaction (from about one-sixth of the establishment-based sample replying) had to do with relationships, not with the staff but with other residents. Here, perhaps, we should note that the 'complainer' might be equally at fault, if fault is the right word. Mr King's wife, acting as his proxy, implied this of her husband.

> Sister said they put him in among the men sooner than expected because the women patients in this hospital rattled him and he doesn't like women. He's a well-known woman-hater. Why he ever wanted to marry, I don't know!

The unacceptable, probably very common, face of communal living was vehemently described by Mr Abbott in talking about another resident: 'She makes me sick and I feel like spewing up everything I've had to eat, the way she coughs. She doesn't cough in an ordinary way, but as if she's going to be sick, and that's why I don't like her.'

Attitudes such as these, however, or at any rate their expression, were the exception in our study. On the whole there appeared to be at the least an acceptance of other people's foibles or shortcomings and at best an ability or willingness to ignore them or, like Mrs Arthur, to take a positive pleasure in the company available.

Feelings about old age

Finally, the replies to a question on their feelings about old age will help to fill out the picture of life satisfaction of very old people. There was wide variation in the replies from very positive ones (of which there were marginally the most), to negative ones. Fewest in number were those showing neutral or uncertain feelings. Thus, in this last category, Mr Symonds was 'not sure if it's a punishment or a reward. It's hard to understand why some people die at 80 and others not.' The thought that he was much older 'never occurred' to Mr Dean until he got our request for his participation in the study. 'Your letter put years on me!' And Mrs Forbes commented that all the people she used to know were dead – 'that makes me feel very old, but ordinarily I don't think about it'.

On the negative side, Mrs Hopkins, with a high level of disability, found

old age very hard to accept. I see nothing at all to recommend it – nothing. I think old age is wicked if you ask me anything. When you are no longer any use in the world it seems to be hopeless to go on living, especially if you have always lived a useful life and someone has been dependent on you.

Mrs Horden, by contrast, thought old age was 'nice': 'It's lovely. I'm very grateful and very happy about it. Rob [her son] says I am going to get a telegram from the Queen. He's a very lovely chap and he's so gentle and thoughtful to old people.'

SUMMARY

In this chapter, carrying forward our discussion in Chapter 5, we have attempted to explore some of the complex and important relationships between the elderly individuals' perceptions of the quality of their everyday life, and the circumstances in which they live.

It is clear from our evidence, that poor health status and severe disability, especially poor mobility, can have a negative effect on the experience of everyday life, though even here there were individuals who had adapted to their restrictions. Health is not the only factor to influence a person's outlook on life; social circumstances also play a part. The presence of strong family ties, for instance, was an important influence. But it must be said that many of the social circumstances and much of the current health status of individuals affect the subjective quality of life in ways which defy 'linear' causal interpretations, particularly where there are as many marked individual variations from the general pattern as were apparent in our sample.

For many in our study, life was approached with serenity and a sense of contentment. The present still held pleasure (even when pastimes were of a 'passive' variety) and the future was contemplated with a sense of inevitability or even 'completeness'. At the least, daily life after 90 need not be characterized by unhappiness. The positive impact of a long and varied life course can often provide a sense of meaning to life even when health and mobility have declined.

Having established these basic contours of daily life, our discussion now needs to take into account issues such as dependency, choice and care. These bring into focus crucial aspects of the quality of life in a wider social context. It is to these issues that we turn in the next two chapters.

7

DEPENDENCY AND CHOICE

Social interaction on a day-to-day level is likely to take on new meaning with advancing age; inevitably, in some respects, its extent for the oldest old will be more limited. This does not mean, however, that self-determination is any less an imperative for them than for younger people.

In this chapter, we consider the possibilities and nature of independence for someone aged 90 or 100 and, in the light of the debate about 'structured dependency', the problems and realities of dependence. In discussing the issue of interdependence and reflecting on the nature of reciprocity, we take note of the help and support given to others by the elderly people of the sample. We examine the significance of responsibility for very old people and look at the kinds of responsibilities carried by members of our sample. We also consider the question of choice as this concerns elderly people's control over daily life, and of possible risks to well-being, or even to life and limb, arising from the circumstances and health status of the individual. All these are considered in the light of the evidence we have on the quality of life at home compared with that of communal life.

INDEPENDENCE AND DEPENDENCE

In asking, as we must, how far full independence for very old people is a maintainable, or even a desirable, goal, a prior question intervenes. What do we mean by independence, or dependence? Elias challenges our common perceptions of dependence as a negative state when he says:

> It is somewhat difficult to convey the depth of the dependence of people on each other; that the meaning of everything a person

118

does lies in what he or she means to others, not only to those now alive but also to coming generations; that she or he is therefore dependent on the continuation of human society through generations is certainly one of the most fundamental of human mutual dependencies.

(Elias 1985:33)

Traditional definitions of dependency that imply a degree of undesirable need are those most likely to be used for very old people. Even if we take a simple definition such as 'a state in which actions by others are a necessary condition for an actor to achieve his or her own goals' (Anderson 1971), the degree of dependence can vary according to the elderly person's capacities and desires. In the same way, the ability or willingness to meet the need on the part of the 'carer' may vary according to their interpretation of the need. 'What', Wenger (1986: 72) asks, 'does *needing* help mean? Does it mean that the task could not be accomplished without help even to save one's life, or does it mean that it is nice to have help because it removes the fear of failing or accomplishes the task more quickly?'

So definitions can obfuscate the issues. More helpful, perhaps, is to focus attention on different kinds of dependence – economic, physical, emotional and social, recognizing that there is inevitably interaction between them.

Technically, it would appear that the status of economic dependence applies to anyone over retirement age. Official 'dependency rates' are calculated on this basis (CSO 1988: Table 1.5). This leads into the whole debate about structured dependency, a term which offers a critical view of the supposed costs and benefits of an ageing population (see e.g. Townsend 1981; Walker 1981, 1983; Macnicol 1990; Townsend 1989). The debate centres on the idea of mandatory or 'enforced' retirement, the presence of poverty, and institutionalization. Since the elderly no longer contribute to the economy and are obliged to rely for their livelihood on state pensions and welfare, the 'marginalization' of the elderly is a product of the social structure rather than an inherent feature of ageing. In turn these processes are obscured by blaming the elderly for being a 'burden'. There are counter arguments to this thesis which rely, among other factors, on the changing age structure of the population, and the effects of welfare provision which may be less of a 'drain' on the productive economy, than a part of a new and growing 'consumer market'. Changing cultural images, notably a diminution in the strength of the work ethic, are also said to play a part in reducing marginalization (Kholi 1988: 384). Likewise, the assumed negative effects of reliance on state support may be misplaced.

Whatever the pros and cons of the debate in general about structured dependency and the elderly, three points need making in relation to very old people. First, as Falkingham (1987: 19) has pointed out, predicted age-related increases in the dependency ratio would seem to have been exaggerated; the growing numbers of the oldest old, economically speaking, will be offset by changes in the labour market, 'including those of falling rates of unemployment and of increasing female labour force participation' (ibid). Secondly, although the boundary between work and retirement, even today and certainly for our study age group, is less sharply drawn for many women than for men, households headed by elderly women living alone (along with those by a lone mother) are most at risk from poverty (Glendenning and Millar 1987), and as we have made clear, women greatly predominate in our age group. Thirdly, the steep rise in communal living among the very old means that residential status should feature prominently in any analysis of dependency in this age group.

Among very old people, at least on the basis of our findings, poverty seems less in evidence. Apart from the fact that the majority belonged to social classes III, II or I, there was also the question of shared incomes (as we assumed) among many living with relatives in private households (and sometimes the addition of an attendance allowance). This in itself, it could be argued, was a form of dependency, though at best, of mutual dependence. Furthermore, high proportions of the sample were in communal establishments where, for many, personal incomes are subsidized.

Another measure of economic dependence we used had to do with control over personal finances. Just under half the total sample replying said that they managed their own money. Among those in private households, however, they formed the majority. The fact that a majority also either owned their homes or were the nominated tenant in itself suggests a fair measure of economic independence. Personal finances, where not managed by the elderly people themselves, were variously looked after by spouses, members of the family or professionals. Mrs Vernon's solicitor, for instance, had power of attorney and Mrs Lipton, living alone, talked of her accountant though she managed her own day-to-day expenditure.

Of those in communal establishments who did not manage their own money, over two-fifths were unable to do so. Information either from the elderly people or from proxies was rather sparse, but where it existed it was possible to detect a difference between the few of some wealth whose financial affairs were managed by independent professionals, solely or together with a member of the family, and those where relatives or staff were responsible, together or separately.

A strong and, in our view, entirely justified case is made in the Wagner Report (1988: 39–40) for individual financial autonomy, where it is feasible, in a communal setting. It does occur, and there were examples among our sample. But also, among fully alert and mentally sound people, there were examples of the opposite. Mr Todd, for instance, in a local authority home, said he 'just had pocket money' and Mrs Cuthbert, in a private home, also spoke of pocket money.

Turning now to other forms of dependency, particularly those concerned with maintaining a degree of autonomy in physical activities, we find again that there are differences according to type of residence. It is also clear that attitudes, both on the part of very old people and of those who may provide support, are an important influence.

Almost inevitably, some physical independence must be relinquished with entry into an establishment, but not necessarily as much as is usually assumed. Much, of course, will depend on the extent of physical or mental disability sustained by the individual. But keeping in mind that this discussion relates to the quality of life, the response to dependency, however caused, will be influenced by the *quality* of the physical or mental care given (see Hughes and Wilkin 1987). In this connection, the question arises of how much independence those running and servicing the establishment are prepared to foster and encourage, and this applies not only to physical dependence but to psychological and social as well. It is also worth noting that a recent study casts doubts on the relevance of such encouragement to the question of dependency (Booth 1986). Other factors, such as 'routinization' and control, the personalities, life experiences, physical health of the residents, staff skills, were thought to have more bearing on the matter than differences between 'a protective model of care or a more supportive [one]' (ibid: 234, 235).

From all this we can see that the diversity among very old people which has been evident whatever aspect of their lives we have considered, is again, both within and between the two main settings, apparent in their degrees of physical and social dependency. We have used the overall disability measure – PDS (see Chapter 4) – to help us assess these varying degrees and relate them to their feelings in the matter. Staying for the moment with those in communal establishments we found considerable contrast in their levels of disability and their attitudes, the two extremes exemplified by Mrs Arthur on the one hand, and Mrs Preston on the other. The former, with her membership of the Womens' Guild, her low level of disability and the 'positive influence' she was said to exert on her fellow residents, maintained considerable independence. Mrs Preston, in a long-stay hospital, was totally deaf, incontinent and in need of constant care, and yet she evinced a relatively cheerful acceptance of her situation. Then there was Mr Baldwin who, when asked if he could manage to do anything for himself, replied, 'Not lately but I do still try – I try to sew my buttons on.' With a high level of disability he had, as had others, strong views about independence, even if he himself could no longer maintain it. 'I think really people should never be sent to these places [long-stay hospitals]. You see they don't do anything for themselves.'

In private households the same diversity was apparent. Mr Morgan, for instance, whose level of disability was well below the norm, lived alone, drove a car 'with an orange badge', and engaged in a variety of leisure activities, but, as the following comments reveal, independence and dependence are often difficult to separate.

> It's the walking that beats me – I use two sticks. When I come out from the Co-op or Marks and Spencers with my groceries I wait on the step outside and catch somebody and ask, 'Would you mind carrying this bag and putting it on the bonnet for me on that little red car?' People are marvellous.

Mrs Warner, with good reason, described herself as 'a very independent lady'. Mrs Fairlie, approaching her hundredth birthday and very frail, was almost wholly dependent on the daughter with whom she lived. She was, nevertheless, 'resigned' to her vanished independence, sustained, it seems, by a deep Roman Catholic faith.

In both settings, distress at the loss of independence was apparent among some members of the sample – witness Mrs Hopkins' despair (see Chapter 6, p. 110) – or fear of losing it, as evidenced by their worries about being a burden. Mr Britton spoke for many:

> As the years go by I do have my anxieties – I cannot see what the future holds for me as I lose my capacity to look after myself. I should hate having to be looked after by somebody else.

Equally, as we have seen, independence was highly valued, and often, as with Mr Ross, fiercely pursued as an objective. In between these extremes of attitude lay the majority whose condition might best be described as semi-dependent. Among these were some who, like Mrs Benson, were sometimes unhappy or, like Mrs Ricketts, deeply unhappy with their present lot. Many, however, seemed content to accept their present position or their probable future progress towards greater dependency – an acceptance set against a life course of effort and supplying support to others.

The substantial minority who seemed quite willing to identify caring activities as such by those designated as carers, illustrates the seemingly untroubled acceptance of the state of some dependency they experienced. Mrs Stubbs, 106 years old and resident in a private rest home, with relatively little disability, perceptively summed up what seemed to her a fair compromise. 'I try not to be too independent. When you come into a place like this, people would like you to be dependent on them and learn to love them – and you get love in return'.

The role of the formal caring services is obviously important for the position of very old people living in the community. We shall be looking at this in Chapter 8.

Whether we take Elias' larger view of dependency as an inherent feature of human life or focus only on the problems that economic and social dependency can create, we may extend our understanding of either view by considering the question of reciprocity.

RECIPROCITY

Gouldner (1960: 161) begins his classic essay on reciprocity with a quotation from Cicero: 'There is no duty more indispensable than that of returning kindness.' Along the road, he suggests that: 'beyond reciprocity as a pattern of exchange and beyond folk beliefs about reciprocity as a fact of life, there is another element: a generalized moral norm of reciprocity which defines certain actions and *obligations* as repayments for benefits received' (ibid: 170). This norm of reciprocity, he later claims, 'cannot apply with full force in relations with children, old people or with those who are physically or mentally handicapped' (ibid: 178).

In his matter-of-fact introduction to exchange theory Bredemeier, (1978: 418) suggests that 'the stability of any set of interdependencies calls for agreement on who does and should exchange what with whom for what reasons and on what terms.' Such agreements are likely to be more difficult to arrive at where Gouldner's excepted groups are concerned than for the generality of society. That 'old people', however, should number among these groups would now be strongly questioned. Both elderly people themselves, together with concerned organizations, are fighting hard for recognition of their actual and potential contribution to society. The contribution can take many forms, not least at the level of family and community care and support.

Moreover, reciprocal acts – gift and counter-gift – need not necessarily be made at the same time. For the elderly (unlike a 'dependent' group such as the mentally handicapped), the element of time is all-important; the notion of credit (Titmuss 1970: 199) may bring comfort to those no longer able to 'be useful'. It would, however, be foolish to deny that general constraints and particular restrictions on such contributions must increase with age.

Being useful suggests practical help; being wanted implies reciprocal acts of love and friendship, of which being useful may be a part. Within the family, very old people may justly consider that the 'credit' of their earlier parental care, financial support and the like, administered over the years, may be reciprocation enough for the current acts of love and support of their children. But this must clearly be seen by the relatives to be a fair exchange. In most cases among our study group this seemed to be the case.

The problem arises when, by any standards, the physical and emotional 'burden' of caring becomes intolerable, where intergenerational tensions in judging credits arise, where the exchange relationship on either side is contaminated by feelings of guilt, remorse, or where dementia interrupts normal exchange. Then, too, it must not be forgotten that a 'vacuum' (Titmuss 1970: 72) may have occurred long ago and may have been filled, if not with hostility and conflict, then with misunderstanding and coolness. There was evidence of both hostility and misunderstanding among members of our sample, but compared with the opposite frame of mind, such feelings belonged very much to the minority.

We asked two questions directly concerned with the idea of interdependence or reciprocity. First, whether there was anyone dependent on them for anything and, secondly, how they felt about the fact that they were doing something, or were no longer able to do anything, for someone else. Over three-quarters of the sample members replying to the first question said no-one was dependent on them. The thirty-eight members of the actual sample replying in the affirmative, were composed of seven of the sixteen married men, and the remaining eleven consisted of men and women of different ages, widowed and single, in a variety of residential settings. The great majority of the examples of reciprocity were in the nature of emotional support or acts of friendship, the recipients of which were variously, relatives, neighbours, friends or fellow residents. 'I have friends', said Mrs Arthur, 'who I know come to me with their problems. Like that I feel I am here for some good.' Additionally, financial help to children was given in nine instances and personal care by the seven husbands to their wives.

The great majority of those giving support to others said that it did help them. But among those who were asked whether no longer being able to do anything upset them, or was reckoned to be 'fair enough', three-quarters expressed the latter view, suggesting that at least among the elderly people there was a recognition of the idea of 'credit'.

Similar questions arise in considering responsibilities, the presence or absence of which may be central to providing a role in daily life.

For most people, in the same way that dependency is likely to increase once the tenth decade is reached, and even earlier, so also there will almost certainly be a diminishing of roles and responsibilities. Younger people may bemoan their responsibilities – as spouse, parent, worker, householder, daughter or son – but would find life strange and, probably, the poorer without them.

The responsibility of running a home either in its day-to-day aspects or, as the 'responsible householder' (often as home owner), has particular relevance to our study in the light of the proportions of our sample still in this position, and also of those living alone. When Mr Rossiter, for example, a childless 96-year-old widower on his own, was asked if he worried about the upkeep of his house he replied, 'I get a bit fed up at times and think about going into a home to avoid it, but then again I can please myself what I do.' Discharging responsibilities is a way of maintaining a strong sense of self-worth.

Just as a considerable measure of independence can be maintained in residential establishments, so responsibility may be a positive and rewarding part of communal life, and a source of social roles provided that it is desired and is not exploited. At the routine level, we found to a limited extent that a variety of small jobs were performed by sample members. At a more exacting level, there was little evidence of participation by the residents in running the place – in staff selection, for instance (see e.g. Wagner 1988: 195), or in the organizing of leisure activities.

Independence, reciprocity and responsibility may help reduce a sense of powerlessness in very old age, but the opportunity for choice, facilitated by favourable material and familial circumstances, and the availability of alternatives, also comes into the picture.

CHOICE

The most obvious 'choice' that arises in very old age concerns that between living in a private household and a communal establishment.

The choice between home and Home

Among any group of individuals, and certainly among the very old, there will inevitably be some, those suffering from senile dementia, for instance, or serious confusion, for whom the question of choice must certainly involve the judgements of others.

Within these limits, the decision to move from 'own home' to a communal establishment should arguably be taken as a 'free' and positive choice (Wagner 1988). But, like all such decisions and situations, this is rarely clear cut. Perhaps the elderly person would prefer to move in with relatives, but senses a reluctance on their part or knows it to be 'impossible'. Either of which sentiments may be justified from the relatives' point of view. In many cases there is a possible conflict of interest between family and individual.

Such a conflict was evident between Mrs Phillips and her daughter, already living together, although there were prospects of its resolution. Mrs Phillips said she spent all her time in her room at the back of the bungalow, feeling isolated. At 92 she was physically independent and reported a number of leisure activities, but despite this felt herself to be a 'burden' and 'intruding' on her daughter's life:

> I'd like to go into a home. I go fortnights to a place I've got my name down for. I could be comfortable there; people of my own age. My daughter wants me to go, though she won't say it. My daughter and her husband are retired and want to go around more, like going to see my granddaughter in Australia, but I feel as though I'm stopping them.

Other factors may act as a barrier to positive choice in favour of such a move – the reputation, for instance, of local public or private establishments, or the non-availability of a place in the one preferred, which was the case with Mrs Benson. Or there was Mr Harker. He had, it seems, been unsuccessful a few years previously in obtaining an 'old person's flat' (after his wife had died) and had run up a lot of bills:

> I went into an Old People's Home to get over it and have a rest.

But it wasn't a rest at all – the noisiest place I've ever been in. I had to share a room with a snorer, among other things.

It is not, however, only those with low levels of disability for whom choice in this respect should be possible. This is where the support of formal caring services are important, as much when the individuals are being cared for by relatives as when they are not, though in the former case the viewpoint of the carers cannot be ignored. If the individual's choice is for staying within the community then the role of the formal providers is now frequently seen as one of *offering* choices rather than *making* them (Anderson and Bury 1988: 2). For the most part, those living in private households made it clear that they were there from choice.

Among those already in communal establishments, our questioning did not go deep enough to uncover possible 'subtle coercion' (Peace 1988: 230) by professionals and family which may have been instrumental in placing them there in the first place. Nor can we be sure that even where there was no coercion the original choice was initiated by the individual. We do know, however, that the majority, at least at the interviewing stage, did not want to move (see Chapter 6).

We know also that for some, genuine choice in entering an establishment had occurred. Mrs Stubbs told her interviewer that six years previously, at the age of 100, she had decided that things at home, particularly the garden, were getting too much for her. On consulting her GP, he had recommended a private residential home just about to be opened in the neighbourhood, and there she had been ever since.

By contrast, there was Mrs Ellis, described by the interviewer as 'most unhappy'. Her freedom of choice had, it seems, been frustrated by her family (an instance, perhaps, of not such subtle coercion, though it is fair to say we did not obtain the family's point of view), who refused to have her at home. She was, according to the interviewer, being kept in a cottage hospital against her will and the doctor's wishes. The hospital staff thought she was totally unsuited to a hospital ward ('too lively and active to be confined') and were frustrated by the family's attitudes. Mrs Ellis kept asking 'Why am I here?'

Choice within the community

Living in the community, then, is still generally considered to be the preferred way of life for most people, as well as a tenet of social policy. Among our sample, many were 'settled', 'happy' or 'contented', were near their families or had good neighbours. A few offered less positive reasons for their choice. They felt they were 'too old to move', were reluctant to give up their own home or their independence, or had 'nowhere better to go'.

By the time an individual reaches the age of 90 the preference may be diluted not only by practical considerations but also by such matters as increased isolation, reluctance to continue the carrying of responsibilities or anxiety about 'being a burden' to relatives. Also, from the relatives' point of view, where it applies, as we have seen with Mrs Phillips' daughter, there are problems intrinsic to their role as carers. Thus, the perceptions of reciprocity and choice significantly change over time.

If, however, an elderly person has opted to remain within the community, there is still a range of choices that may be open to them. Some, such as Mr Compton, had chosen to live with relatives – with their full agreement. The choice of living alone was for many sample members still apparently a free one, especially if, as with Mrs Johnson, a devoted family lived nearby. Mrs Chester's position illustrates certain of the dilemmas attaching to a range of choices. She, at the age of 96, in good health and described by her interviewer as *very* independent, had chosen to live alone in a purpose-built flat attached to her son and daughter-in-law's house. Despite her stated concern not to rely on her family she nevertheless expressed worries during the interview at 'being a burden' and at the fact that she might be holding her son and daughter-in-law back from taking more or longer holidays. She was even wondering whether she should 'go into a home'.

Mrs Baines, aged 98, on the other hand, exercising her freedom to choose, unsubjected to pressure, did not intend leaving her privately rented terrace house, lacking in all mod. cons. A few, like Mrs Latham, living alone in a detached house and fortunate in her financial situation, wished for something more convenient – 'a small bungalow without a garden but with a warden'. So she was about to choose sheltered housing.

The small group of our sample members already in sheltered housing appeared to be there from choice, with every intention, if possible, of remaining there. Whether this would ultimately prove feasible, we are not in a position to say.

Very old people, it seems, are much less likely to be in sheltered housing than the young elderly (see e.g. Hunt 1978: Table 8.2.1; Middleton 1987: 28) found only five women who were aged 90 or over. In an OPCS survey (Hunt 1978) only 5·4 per cent of the total were aged 85 and over. The corollary of these low proportions is likely to be that a 'move into sheltered housing is not infrequently followed by a second move into a residential establishment, because of the difficulty of maintaining and increasing the levels of support which become necessary' (Wagner 1988: 20).

Our seven sheltered housing individuals had been resident for between two and nine years. They mostly had relatively low levels of disability, though some had difficulty with stairs and only two went out without help. For two there were doubts about the advisability of their staying; in Mrs Woods' case a move was being pressed for by her daughter against her mother's wishes.

For the remaining five, there was unanimity of opinion among the elderly residents, the 'carers' (in most cases wardens or housemothers), and the interviewers about the suitability of their living arrangements, and for none did a move seem imminent or desirable; quite the reverse. This does not necessarily invalidate the supposition that second moves are likely, since we have no evidence about the frequency of moving among other very old residents, both past and present.

In concentrating on choice concerning *where* people live, we do not intend to underestimate the importance of choice concerning *how* people live. Freedom of choice in such everyday matters as what to have for breakfast and when to have it, whether or not to watch the telly, which clothes to put on, shading into those areas of choice that carry risk, is a crucial element in the concept of dependency and, indeed, in the personal relationships which are central to it. Our data suggest that many of those both living alone and with others in private households, had a considerable amount of such freedom, even where there was a fair degree of dependency, though clearly the range of choice was to some extent contingent upon other factors in their everyday lives.

Choice within communal establishments

In Muriel Spark's *Momento Mori*, Miss Taylor, suffering under the 'lacerating familiarity of the nurses' treatment' in the early stages of her sojourn in the 'Maud Long Medical Ward (aged people, female)' taught herself to bear the 'desolate humiliation' by 'resolving to make her suffering a voluntary affair'. Thereby she gained 'a decided and visible dignity' (Spark 1959: 10). Thus in one sense she was exercising some form of countervailing power, though the basis upon which it relied was by any standards an unacceptable one.

At a less shocking and more practical level, there is, or should be, within the communal setting, room for some freedom of choice, even in hospitals, as can be found, for example, in The Bolingbroke Hospital (Millard 1985) and St Pancras Hospital (Rastan 1989), both in London. The fact that someone has chosen to go into residential care, or, even more so if they have been placed there against their preference, should not mean that, once there, they relinquish all further choice, any more than that their dignity be undermined.

In their study of physical care in residential homes, Hughes and Wilkin (1987:410) found only one member of staff who gave residents 'a choice as to *when* they would like to bathe'. So choice may centre on tending activities – whether, indeed, these are always necessary, and by whose judgement – and on the manner in which they are carried out. But the question of choice for the individual resident arises in other matters – in companionship and relationships, in the practicalities of daily living, in the disposition of their belongings, in the extent of privacy, in the range of leisure activities, in opportunities for participation in running the establishment.

Finally we should note that choice also involves risk, a matter which has received some attention in recent discussions of the quality of life of the elderly (Norman 1980; Brearly 1982).

RISK

This discussion has challenged paternalistic views about risk among old people, especially the assumption that old age must not be accompanied by risk. Our own study shows that avoiding all risks is not always the highest priority. Risks presuppose rights – the right to take risks (Norman 1980). The question, therefore, is how much risk for extremely old, possibly frail, people is acceptable and whose definition of risk should prevail? By phrasing the question thus, the implication is that others – officialdom and relatives – have the right, even the duty, to intervene, and in certain ways restrict the individual's freedom of choice, thereby reducing or eliminating risk. This, inevitably, has consequences for that person's independence, which brings us back to the question whether in fact 'rights to risk' do diminish with the loss of responsibilities in very old age. If, however, there is a 'right' of intervention by others, is there not also a right of individual elderly people to live in squalor if they want to, to shun help in crossing the road, to continue living on the first floor even if it means having to crawl up and down stairs, or, like Mr Unwin, to drive a car against his family's wishes?

It is true that some of these activities involve risk to others, though this applies right through the life course. Equally, even where there is no risk to others, there are ways of reducing risk while preserving at least some independence. In the institutional setting, for instance, there is a world of difference between tactful supervision and carefully worked-out rules governing care and attendance and the wholesale imposition of control and intervention.

The main problem lies in the assumption that age itself is the determining factor and that very old age requires a special set of values and practices to be 'imposed', however 'tactfully', by others. Indeed, irrespective of whether the elderly person lives within the community or in an establishment, what is needed above all is a shift in underlying attitudes 'away from a patronizing and paternalistic over-protection from risk towards acknowledgement of their right to as much self-determination as is possible for each individual within the limits of the resources available' (Norman 1980:8).

Regardless of underlying attitudes, however, there is a difference between acceptable risks and tolerable risks (Brearley 1982: 47). Some people tolerate risks which are unacceptable by normally recognized standards because they are powerless to affect the situation (ibid) or, we would add, because of what some might consider a perverse disinclination to take the easy way out. Either way the degree of *tolerable* risk diminishes with age in inverse proportion to the likelihood of an increase in unacceptable risk. Likewise, the need to monitor degrees of risk increases with age, and it is no accident that 'the very old' constitute a 'risk group' (WHO 1977). We return to this subject in Chapter 8.

Meanwhile, we touch on two further sides to risk and very old people. First, what increases or reduces the possibility of risk, and second, upon what premises are decisions involving the possible reduction or intensification of risk taken. It is, for instance, generally assumed that entry into residential care will reduce risk. This view has been questioned. If people are already at risk, moving them out of their homes may not reduce the risk – indeed the prognosis is that it may become worse (Norman 1980: 17). On the second point, to what extent is a decision taken purely in the self-perceived interests of the elderly person? How much, for example, is the 'solution' of moving in with children to the advantage of the elderly person or a matter of meeting the relative's anxieties and guilt feelings (ibid:23)? Certainly, if the proportions of our sample members still living alone mean anything they indicate that a good many people aged 90 and over in England today may be prepared to take risks for the sake of independence.

SUMMARY

While we would not wish to underestimate 'dependency needs' amongst the very old, including the needs for physical and emotional care which were evident in our survey, we have argued in this chapter that concepts such as 'reciprocity', 'credit' and 'choice' are essential to an understanding of the meaning of dependency in very old age.

It is clear that very old age does involve a loss of responsibilities in terms of social roles. As Riley *et al.* (1988) have recently pointed out, this is a major source of dependency. Such loss of roles, however, invites a view of the elderly person in terms of biological or physiological age characteristics alone. It also underpins the popular view that very old age involves a return to the dependency of childhood. Hence the tendency to refer to old people in child-like terms.

We suggest, in contrast, that dependency should be seen as an unavoidable feature of the quality of life at any age, involving complex dynamics of choice and constraint. This more 'realist' perspective would move us away from assuming that dependency can always be overcome, and towards a recognition that, under some circumstances, especially with advancing years, it might bring some benefits to the individual. Whilst the loss of autonomy and social responsibilities can mean distress and difficulty, this is not always the case. In regarding dependency as containing positive as well as negative components, essential features not only of old age but also of social life in general may be discerned.

In this, as in other areas of the quality of life, we have constantly touched on the importance of social relationships and social support in very old age. We deal with this issue more fully in the next chapter.

8

SUPPORT AND CARE

In this chapter, we explore further the dynamics of independence, dependence, reciprocity, and the rights and obligations of very old people in their relationships with those closest to them – family, neighbours and friends on whom they may count for support and very often, care. We examine the influences that these relationships have on the quality of their lives.

We have attempted to draw a distinction between support and care, as others have before us. Bulmer (1987: 19, 20), for instance, developing Parker's (1981) distinction between two types of care in the community, contrasts the 'hard end' of informal care, which consists mainly of 'tending' activities such as feeding, washing, lifting, cleaning up the incontinent, protecting and comforting, with 'less burdensome forms of care which do not involve actual physical contact with the person being cared for'. But they do, of course, involve social contact. These latter kinds of care, or what we have chosen to call support, arguably make fewer demands on relatives and friends, and pose fewer mutual problems, but they have both material and psychological components (Bulmer 1987). In the present study, family and friends gave some kind of informal support to members of the sample living in communal establishments as well as in private households, and our discussion will take both of these into account.

A consistent theme of this book has been the significance of the life course for the changes and continuities in the lives of very old people. For the topic of this chapter its relevance is doubly strong, since the life course of the supporters and carers is also of account, in that they themselves are likely to be entering old age, or have already reached it, with changing expectations and obligations.

We begin by identifying the potential supporters and the frequency of contact between them and the individuals in our study. We next discuss the kind of support that was given and how it was valued by the sample members. In the second part we move on to the subject of care. First, following Abrams (1984), we focus within the community, on the informal carers and cared-for and on formal care – the part played by the professional caring services. Secondly, we consider care within communal establishments.

INFORMAL SUPPORT NETWORKS

Contact with families

At each stage of the life course, the individual is enmeshed in 'a variety of kinship and social groups, all of which bring interactions and relationships with family, friends and neighbours' (Victor 1987: 213). Towards the end of a very long life, these groups may begin to disintegrate. The members of our sample, however, despite their great age, were, for the most part, still firmly enmeshed, at least in a kinship network. Spouses, as we have seen, had mostly died but other kin, even though partially depleted, were strongly in evidence.

Twenty-two per cent of the total sample, including the single, were known to have had no children. Of those who had, and here we include individuals such as Miss Gregory and her adopted daughters,the great majority of the children were still living, most of whom were married. Thirty-five per cent of the total sample had had families of three or more children, of whom more than half had had five or more.

Having children does not necessarily mean that there is a bond with them. Furthermore, such a bond, if it exists, may wither if the opportunity to maintain it is denied, though in these days of the telephone, children living at a distance of fifty miles or more (or even in different continents) may still maintain a close relationship. Abrams (1988: 63), while recognizing that an increasing number of elderly people are living alone, makes the positive point that technology and higher real incomes now '[provide] the elderly with new opportunities for social contact'. Very old people, however, may find using the fruits of technology difficult and, in fact only 46 per cent of the total sample used the telephone, or had access to one. We have also (in Chapter 4) seen that writing letters was an infrequent occurrence.

These problems, however, affected only a small minority where their children were concerned, since very few had children living beyond a radius of fifty miles. The majority – 65 per cent, including the substantial minority who were actually living with their children – had one or more child within a distance of five miles, a proportion

Table 8.1 Frequency of contact with relatives (other than spouse): weighted
           sample

Frequency of contact	Total %
Never	2.6
Less than monthly	11.9
At least once a month	12.0
At least once a week	33.7
(Almost) daily	24.2
Lives with	15.5
Total	100[1]
	(192)

[1]See note 2.

approximating to that of other findings related to the elderly (see e.g.
Victor 1987: 221).

We are concerned with a long-lived group of people with a
relatively high proportion of long-lived siblings. Grandchildren and
great grandchildren, nephews and nieces also figured in the kinship
network, many of whom, together with numbers of children, gave
support. If we include those who were living with various relatives,
two-fifths of the total sample saw one or other of them (almost) every
day, and a further third at least once a week (see Table 8.1).

Discounting the group who were living with relatives, daily contact
with family occured twice as often among those in private households
as among those in communal establishments – for roughly two-fifths of
the former compared with just over one-fifth of the latter (see Table A
2.13). The fact, however, that daily contact of one kind or another was
more frequent among the domiciliary group was, to some extent, offset
among the establishment group by a higher proportion among them of
weekly and monthly encounters. It seems clear from this that family
bonds, even if in a more attenuated form, continue through what might
be termed the barrier of institutionalization.

The relative frequency with which our sample members saw their
families is in line with that of many earlier and more recent studies of
elderly people in the community (see e.g. Townsend 1957; Abrams
1978; Bowling *et al.* 1988) and, further, tends to counteract the evidence
that among the very old there is an apparent decline in 'overall contact
with family members' (Victor 1987: 222).

135

The never-marrieds are commonly held to be 'much less likely to have family contacts than either the married or the widowed' (ibid). This proportionately was not the case among our sample. Nephews, nieces, brothers, sisters and cousins often filled the vacuum in terms of contact, though a higher proportion than among the widowed were to be found in communal establishments. But, central though family ties are, it is not only relatives who can provide help and companionship.

Neighbours and friends

Contact with people other than family has especial relevance for those who have no living relatives or never see them – a mere 3 per cent of the total sample, only seven members of the actual sample. Even among these small numbers, as elsewhere, diversity was apparent, comprising as they did women and men, widowed and single, childless and those who had had children (two), some living in communal establishments (the majority) and some in private households.

Temperament, behaviour, attitudes and the 'compensation' of contact with friends or neighbours also varied among this small group without relatives. Mrs James, referred to by the 'key worker' of her residential home as 'the grandmother I never had', was cheerful and active, with friends she saw regularly. Mrs Dodds, living alone in a sheltered housing unit, relied on three ex-neighbours for support. Mrs Hopkins, according to the matron, 'usually started the day in tears', but was supported by several friends.

Mr Dale was friendless; Mr Hampton, aged 100, also. Described by the matron of his home as 'awkward and bloody-minded', he was clearly unhappy. Mr Dickens, by contrast, who had lived for 52 years with a companion who had originally come to look after his wife, was cheerful, very active and saw seven neighbours at least once a week.

Taking all those living in private households – with or without family – as many as 44 per cent said that they saw no neighbours at home. This relatively large proportion has particular force in view of the generally high proximity of neighbours among our sample – for 93 per cent of those in private households they were living next door. If encounters outside the home are taken into account there was more contact with neighbours; two-fifths of the sample talked of daily or almost daily contact, though it was usually simply a matter of greeting.

Neighbours may well 'qualify' as friends but it makes sense to consider friends separately from neighbours, partly because we must here include those living in communal establishments, and also because for people aged 90 and over, the friendship network is likely to be affected by their present position in the life course. Long-lived women and men do not necessarily have long-lived friends; as indeed, for many, proved to be the case.

'All my friends have gone' was a frequent cry. Nevertheless, although over two-fifths of the private household sample, and just over half of those in establishments said they no longer had any friends, about one-fifth altogether spoke of five or more friends. Information on the frequency of contact was rather sparse, but, of those replying, half of each group said they saw their friends at least once a week. Those living alone saw them considerably more often than others.

The nature of the support

Although simply seeing or being in contact with family, neighbours or friends does not necessarily imply support, among our sample it mostly did, though not always enough, as we saw in Chapter 6, to alleviate feelings of loneliness. In passing we may note that the person most often seen was not always the one most highly valued. Mr Proctor, for instance, was visited regularly by one of his granddaughters, who shopped for him, and for her aunt, his daughter, who, by a happy (or contrived?) coincidence, lived in the same residential home. Father and daughter had their meals together and were clearly on good terms, though it was the granddaughter and her father, Mr Proctor's son, who 'meant most' to Mr Proctor. Mrs Trevor depended on her neighbour for support, but specified her daughter as the most important person.

Under the umbrella of 'support', the elderly people tended to interpret or describe a whole range of practical activities – what Bulmer calls 'material support' (Bulmer 1987: 20). Such were the performance of household chores, help with the garden, generally keeping an eye on things, shopping, collecting the pension, help with knitting or sewing and so on. Not surprisingly, proportionately more of these kinds of activities were undertaken for people living in private households, particularly if living alone, than for those in communal establishments, though in general it was evident that the latter group received a good amount of such support.

In reality, the boundaries between support and care are often ambiguous and vary according to how roles are subjectively perceived. Some intimate household chores, cleaning the toilet, for instance, particularly when contrasted with many external activities, have many personal connotations and their performance merges into the caring role. Both the supporter/carer and the beneficiary may find it difficult to differentiate between practical and emotional kinds of support.

Although the various supporting activities were undertaken mainly by members of the family, neighbours, as we have seen, were also a source of support, particularly where the sample members were living alone. In one or two instances, as we shall see, the neighbours took on a 'caring' role, but in the main they acted more as 'supporters'. Because of the wide-ranging nature of our interest in people aged 90 and over, questions on this topic had to be limited. It does seem, however, that as sources of practical help or just of regular contact – coming in for a chat and similar activities – neighbours were mentioned less often than in some other surveys (e.g. Abrams 1978; Wenger 1984; Sinclair *et al.* 1984). Where there was a close relationship, it was much valued. Mr Waghorn, for instance, spoke with feeling of his next-door neighbour:

> She comes in and offers to do things or brings me things in. When my sister died she did all the running about for me. Nothing is too much trouble. I only have to tap on the wall and she would come straight away.

Mrs Trevor's relationship with her next-door neighbour was characterized by a sense of companionship and friendship. They spent 'several hours a day' chatting together. The interviewer thought that Mrs Trevor, who lived alone, managed well, but 'could be in trouble if the neighbour didn't keep an eye on her'. This was despite regular help and visits from her daughter, her son-in-law, from friends and from the district nurse and a home help; an example of a successful concerted informal and formal effort to keep a very old individual living in the community.

'External' forms of support such as outings – being taken for a drive or on a shopping expedition – were highly prized though they were comparatively rare. Mr Craddock, it may be remembered, lived alone. His daughter told the interviewer that when she and her husband went to 'the Salvation Army we automatically take him with us, though we're going to have a day out on our own this Saturday. If we go out for an evening he very often comes as well.'

Proportionately, however, the most often mentioned, and most highly valued, kind of informal support was that we have categorized as social and emotional. This was sometimes simply a matter of chat or talk, or just the fact of a visit. After all, visiting can be the active expression of interdependence experienced throughout the life course; of valuing and being valued.

All the communal-establishment residents replying to the question said that their (main) visiting relative or friend gave some kind of emotional support. Among those in private households, it was those living alone who proportionately mentioned it most often. Sometimes the reciprocal relationship fostered by the support seemed to go much deeper. Individuals referred to their 'wonderful' daughter or son, saying that they relied on them for 'everything'. This did, of course, in many instances, imply care – or 'tending' activities, to which we now turn.

CARE IN THE COMMUNITY

Compared with support, the notion of care is more closely related to the theme of dependency in the sense of meeting basic needs, and, indeed, to that of independence since the rejection of care, either in fact or in spirit, signals at the very least a desire for independence. Indeed, in accepting care there can also be risks of a loss of power (Bury 1988).

The informal carers

In considering the role of carers, we must remind the reader that although we draw on material from the carer questionnaires, the focus of our study is on the elderly people. Our main concern is with care as it affected those receiving – or not receiving – it. This emphasis by no means implies that we are unaware of the impact of their role on the carers themselves, and we do to a limited extent touch on this in what follows. Full justice to the subject, however, requires a study to itself.

The problem of isolating 'care' from 'support' is compounded in the present study by the fact that we wished to interview people closely connected with our respondents and we made an assumption that theirs would be a caring, or even a 'tending' role. So, in many instances, it was – to a greater or a lesser degree – but sometimes to no degree at all; contact really only entailed 'support' and not invariably even that.

We interviewed seventy-four carers who 'belonged' to the actual sample of eighty-nine people living in private households. In most cases where there was no carer interviewed, it was because the interviewer, for various reasons, could find no appropriate person. A handful of the elderly people objected to such an interview for reasons not always clear. Sometimes, as in Mr Patel's case, it seemed to be a question of the invasion of his privacy. He was himself prepared to give an interview but was deeply worried at the idea that we should talk to anyone else, and required written, as well as verbal, assurances that we respect his wishes.

Sometimes it was a question of the elderly person sharing – explicitly or implicitly – the particular interviewer's assumption that an individual did not have, or need, a 'carer'. This was particularly so with Mr Waghorn. Although he received much 'support' from an affectionate neighbour, 'care' was another matter. Single, aged 95, an ex-pressworker, he lived with a niece who was suffering from ulcerated legs, whom *he* looked after: 'There are plenty of things to do – I do everything around the house – but I sleep well and feel like singing when I get up. When I'm tired I just go to bed and sleep.'

Occasionally, as in the case of Mrs Chester and Mr Lightfoot, the interviewer rejected the idea of such an interview as 'insulting' in the light of the elderly person's obvious ability to look after herself or himself.

These interviewing difficulties illustrate the problem of defining care and the meaning attached to terms such as 'carer'. In current public debate and media interest the category of 'carers' is in danger of becoming reified. Just as 'the elderly' have been treated in the aggregate, 'carers' themselves are grouped together in ways which may have some uses (drawing attention to *their* needs, for example), but which carry the danger of creating a new set of stereotypes. Who is to say, for example, that Mrs Chester's, or Mr Lightfoot's, ability to look after themselves was any greater than Mr Anderson's or Mrs Johnson's, for whom carers were identified? All four individuals lived alone, happy in the 'support' of their respective families or neighbours; none, on the face of it, in need of 'tending' or 'caring' as such.

But to return to those who were interviewed as carers. For those living in private households, children by far outnumbered any other single group (see Table 8.2).

Nine of the elderly men relied on their wives and one or two on their sisters. Mr Russell, at the age of 93, was cared for by his 82-year-old sister, with whom, together with a 92-year-old brother, he lived. She coped with his considerable disabilities (willingly and cheerfully, it seemed), without the help of any professional service.

The great majority of these carers, as we already know, were women. Except for the handful of 'caring' husbands, even where the elderly person was living with a son or nephew, it turned out, in nearly every case, that it was the daughter-in-law or niece-in-law who did the looking after. There was some evidence, as we shall see – mostly

Table 8.2 The informal carers of subjects by sex: weighted sample in private households

Carer	Women %	Men %	Total %
Spouse	0.6	26.3	6.3
Child	58.3	47.4	55.7
Sibling/other relative	8.3	10.5	8.9
Friend/neighbour	15.0	5.3	12.7
Other, e.g. housekeeper, warden of sheltered housing unit, social worker	18.3	10.5	16.4
Total	100[1]	100	100
	(60)	(19)	(79)

[1]See note 2.

implicit rather than explicit – to suggest that this female bias in the caring role was not invariably acceptable.

The informal caring

In answer to a question about how much time they spent in caring, only three carers spoke of a twenty-four-hour job. Yet several, when elaborating on their role, made it clear that they gave total care. The activities described by fifteen carers belonged to the full range within the 'tending' category referred to earlier. Ninety-four-year-old Mr Eastwood's wife was one such. Aged 79, she tended him night and day, washing and dressing him, 'doing everything', though she had occasional visits from a district nurse, weekly visits from a minister of religion and, from friends, help with household chores and with cutting the grass. Mrs Thornton's daughter, aged 72, with whom she lived, also did 'everything', an attendance allowance easing the financial position.

Mrs Singer was partially blind, totally deaf, had a very severe heart condition, bad arthritis and problems of incontinence. She lived with her daughter, aged 57, and son-in-law. The daughter spoke uncomplainingly of the great amount of care she gave her mother, but both she and her husband were resentful of the lack of support coming from other members of the family who lived nearby. An auxiliary nurse gave her mother a weekly bath; the district nurse came occasionally.

As many as twenty-eight carers said that they spent most of their day

– anything between six and eight hours – in caring activities, a large part of an individual's waking life. It is hardly surprising that this was sometimes resented. Some tending activities were carried out by this group, as well as practical tasks – household chores, cooking, washing, shopping and so on. Mr Grainger, for instance, living alone, was visited daily by his daughter who spent four hours (split) in caring and practical activities – shopping, darning, cutting his hair, preparing meals which she would leave for him to put in the oven so as to 'encourage his independence'. A home help and a neighbour made it possible for her to take a holiday, though organizing things for her period of absence 'exhausted' her.

The practical tasks were often conceived by the carers as a form of care, rather than support, even where they were the only activities undertaken. This underlines our earlier point about the weakness of the boundaries between support and care and about the difference between subjective evaluations and objective circumstances. Among the elderly people, there was no reluctance to identify care as such – nearly half of those in private households did so. This showed that despite the fact that the majority thought themselves relatively fit, they seemed untroubled by the notion of care in the specific sense in which we have defined it.

Whether the caring tasks or activities are relatively straightforward or complex and demanding, how the carers and cared-for perceive each other is clearly of importance to an understanding of informal care.

Informal carers and cared-for: mutual perceptions

Where there were expressions of peaceable, warm relationships on one side – of admiration, perhaps, by the carer, of gratitude on the part of the cared-for – these were almost always echoed by the other, and often confirmed by the interviewer, as far as such an assessment may be relied upon. The relationship of Mr and Mrs Eastwood, for instance, was described by the interviewer as 'quite beautiful. They love each other; he knows he needs her and she enjoys being able to care for him.'

The interviewers assessed the majority (well over half) of the relationships between carers and those they were caring for as 'loving' or 'devoted', '(very) good', 'happy, amicable', 'showing mutual respect and affection' and so on, though we recognize that such judgements, made on a single visit, may reflect a desire by the interviewees to demonstrate a positive public face of good family life. A positive relationship existed between Mrs Weston and her daughter, who did 'everything' for her mother, 'there's nothing she can do herself, but she appreciates it all and takes nothing for granted'. Mrs Weston described her daughter as 'marvellous'. Mr Harris was, according to the interviewer, 'completely enveloped' by his family. He lived with one son aged 56, who – unusually – was his main carer, but all the rest (nine surviving out of twelve) lived locally and kept in constant touch. 'They can't do enough', he told the interviewer. 'They do favours for me, talk over old times, keep me company, make sure I've got everything I need.' The son, with whom Mr Harris lived, 'would not dream of letting him go anywhere else'.

Just over two-thirds of the carers said there were no problems or none but minor ones. In answer to a further question, similar proportions said that they suffered no major stress or strain as a result of their caring role. Sometimes, they wished they 'could do more' or were full of praise and gratitude for the uncomplaining nature of the elderly person they were caring for. They were 'very happy to be doing it'. Mrs Vernon's niece, for instance, giving 'total care' to her stone-deaf, poor-sighted, arthritic 100-year-old aunt, expressed admiration and affection for her, an affection, as was clear from the interview, Mrs Vernon herself returned with gratitude. Her nephew-in-law, it seems, sometimes thought that the rest of the family were neglected, but her niece would not contemplate her aunt's transfer to a home.

There were a few carers who thought of what they did as a duty. Mrs King, for instance, said of her husband

> He had a queer idea of life but I lived with him and I had to live his life. After the war I promised – and being a true Quaker you never break a promise – I would always look after him, it didn't matter how old he got or how poorly he got or whatever was the matter with him. Well I did that right until a couple of weeks ago when he went into hospital.

Feelings of emotional strain, physical exhaustion, resentment at the restrictions on their family, occasionally working, lives, and even hostility, or simply neutrality were expressed by an important minority of carers. They felt 'desperate' or just simply needed a break. The case of Mrs Cross, aged 95, who, it may be remembered was incontinent and lived in a house with deficient plumbing, illustrates the significance of the life course for the chief of her two 'caring' daughters, who spent all but two hours of the day with her mother. Her husband had just retired

– a time when he would have welcomed the presence of his wife during the day. Although Mrs Cross lived with her son, her two daughters also (unwillingly) took it in turns to sleep in at night. Mr Weston's daughter, on the other hand, in admitting her need for a break - 'being quite honest, at times, yes. My husband and I love to go to dances and on holiday, but that's finished more or less' – nevertheless added 'but I couldn't leave her and wouldn't want to.'

Mr Crawford has appeared quite often in these pages. Possessing an exceptionally low disability score, his own remarks, and indeed some of those quoted earlier by his daughter-in-law, have shown him to be a man with strong views and independence of spirit, and regarded with some affection by his daughter-in-law. Here, things take on a slightly different complexion. The interviewer described the relationship as 'reasonable'. Nevertheless, she thought that the main drawback seemed to be his deafness which, according to his daughter-in-law,

> makes him boom out whatever he is saying as if he were in the pulpit or delivering a lecture. He's so dictatorial and dogmatic. I cook his meals for him, for which he always thanks God but never me. When he gets up in the morning he booms out prayers of thanks to God for bringing him safely through another night. He also used to sing hymns at night but I had to stop that.

The fact that they were a three-generation household – Mr Crawford, his 66-year-old daughter-in-law and 40-year-old step-granddaughter – did not, it seems, help. Mr Crawford, on the other hand, told the interviewer that he was 'waited on hand and foot' and wished he could do more. Three-generation households may often cause problems. Mr Pratt's daughter-in-law was worried at the 'depressing' effect on her daughter of her father-in-law's condition following a severe stroke. Mrs Chadwick, on the other hand, judging from remarks from both sides, lived with her son, daughter-in-law and granddaughter in complete harmony.

Despite problems and tensions, there was an evident reluctance by nearly all the carers to consider the possibility of permanent alternative arrangements. The largest single group of carers replied with an unequivocal 'no'. Most felt, like Mr Weston's daughter, that they could cope; a small number refused to consider such a move, in spite of difficulties, because it would be 'fatal', or they (the carers) would worry too much.

The 'alternative arrangements' proposed for an individual such as Mr Potter, however, would, it could be assumed, prove satisfactory on both sides. His daughter told the interviewer that her husband was retiring the day after the interview, and they were all planning to move back to a purpose-built house where Mr Potter used to live, as there would be more facilities for care of the elderly when they go on holiday.

Four carers thought those they were looking after would be better off in a home or hospital. Mrs Braithwaite's niece was glad that her aunt was now in hospital after she had collapsed six weeks previously. 'She's much happier there than in her bungalow, which she didn't like.' The relationship between Mrs Phillips and her daughter, seemed to embody a classic case of reluctant caring, with the added twist that the daughter, who shared her mother's desire for a move, apparently felt no guilt about her feelings, only resentment at the present arrangement. This very much seemed to rub off from her husband, who went 'to the pub every lunch time to get out of the house'.

The various feelings about caring – commitment, devotion, sacrifice, guilt, remorse, resentment – touched on here are not new phenomena. When, however, we compare present times with the beginning of this century, for instance, there is a new circumstance. Then, non-familial support for the informal carer came, if at all, from charities, ladies bountiful or servants. Today, there are the formal caring services, statutory and voluntary, where commitment is based on professionalism.

Formal caring services in the community

Domiciliary services

The fact that support from the relevant formal caring services – professional and voluntary – increases with age (see Introduction) gives credence to the view that such support plays a vital part in enabling elderly people, particularly the very old, to stay within the community. As Table 8.3 shows, of our sample members living in private households and replying to this question, significantly the greater proportion received some help, though just under one-quarter (none of whom had any paid help) reported that they were receiving no visits from a district nurse, a home help, a health visitor or meals-on-wheels. Half of those living alone were in this category, which may reflect the relatively good health and the high degree of independence of this group. It also suggests as was found by Evandrou et al. (1986) that there is considerable reliance on the informal carers.

Table 8.3 Support from selected formal care services by who living with: weighted sample in private households

Visits from:	Subject lives		
district nurse, home help, meals-on-wheels or	*alone*	*with others*	*total*
health visitor	%	%	%
Some	66.3	87.3	76.7
None	33.7	12.7	23.3
Total subjects	100	100	100
	(49)	(48)	(97)

There were visits, of course, varying in frequency and regularity, from other individuals, belonging to the various statutory, voluntary and religious agencies – social workers, chiropodists, ministers of religion and so on, but the two key visitors were the district nurse and the home help. Thirty-five per cent, for instance, of all those living in private households were visited at least weekly by a district nurse, and 53 per cent by a home help. Nine per cent saw the district nurse on six to seven days a week, and 32 per cent had a home help on from two to five days.

Although there was an important minority who were not receiving formal help from the key services, it must be said that, as we have seen in some of the illustrations earlier, where there was an obvious need for a formal caring service, this was forthcoming. Where there was no formal support from the health or personal social services, only a few of the informal carers mentioned the need for such visits, either regularly or occasionally. In the case of Mrs Holland, the interviewer wondered if her daughter refrained from asking for help, or medication to relieve her mother's pain, 'in case other members of the family thought she was taking the easy way out by having her mother drugged'.

One or two of the elderly individuals themselves refused to have a home help or meals-on-wheels. With Mrs Locke, this caused serious problems. She was alone during the day, her son staying in the house overnight. Her daughter, who was interviewed as the carer, drove a distance of about seventy miles to see her mother once a week, bringing clean washing, cleaning the house and doing some shopping while she was there. 'It's all a mental drain – even thinking about it is tiring. I can't do any more – I have obligations to my own family.' Mrs Horden referred to the fact that home helps are 'not allowed' to do various things and said that she herself generally did it again next day. 'But you've got to be thankful for small mercies', she continued, 'so you'd better say that it's all right'.

Nearly all the elderly people, however, said that they were content with the provision of services, both in quantity and quality, expressing very high levels of satisfaction . Of the actual sample, there was only one expression of outright dissatisfaction – with the meals-on-wheels service. Otherwise there were occasional gentle complaints or 'mixed feelings' and a few were 'fairly' rather than 'very' satisfied. In all this we are once more reminded of the possibility of an unwillingness by very elderly people to complain, but there was also nothing in the carers' remarks to give an impression of dissatisfaction. We do not know either whether fewer of those already in communal establishments at the time of the interview might have been enabled to stay in the community had more adequate professional support been forthcoming.

As in all matters to do with elderly people and their quality of life, the issue of formal support is not clear cut. Their 'wide variety of needs does not correspond to the relatively inflexible and limited range of services available' (Challis and Davies 1988). In other words, we cannot be sure whether the lack of services amongst our sample should be regarded as a sign of a low level of need, inadequate or unimaginative services or a deliberate choice to do without. We think probably all three, implicit in mutual low expectations, in the uncertainties surrounding the goal of service delivery and a determined resistance to anything suggesting dependency or being categorized as 'poor'. It does, however, seem to support the view that 'community care is a euphemism for family care' (Evandrou et al. 1986). At the time of writing, there is little clarity in government thinking as embodied in the NHS and Community Care Act 1990 (Land in press).

Respite care

As well as the domiciliary services, for frail elderly or handicapped people, another form of professional support may be found in the provision of what is known as respite, or phased, care. It is provided, always with nursing care, by a range of different establishments, for periods of varying length, though usually for two weeks. Seventy per cent of our sample living in private households had never had any respite care; 18 per cent had been into some establishment once, and 12 per cent more than once. Where there are the appropriate facilities, a period of respite care, ideally, enables assessment and reassessment of the patient's condition and, where necessary, treatment. At the same time, it is aimed at giving relief to carers, but as such is not always appreciated by the elderly individual in question. Mrs Trevor who had had one spell of respite care, did not want another. Mrs Nisbett, on the other hand, had found it so satisfactory that she wanted to make a permanent move there from her daughter and son-in-law's home.

Of those who had not experienced it, the great majority said they did not want to. Mr Vincent was one. His feelings were shared by his daughter, despite her 'lack of sleep'. 'He groans in his sleep and also when he's awake.' She listened out for this in the night and checked on her father in case he was in pain. She had not considered alternative arrangements as she felt he was better off with her than in hospital, as she was sure 'he'd starve to death' (he had not, she said, eaten solid food for eight months).

Unwillingness, then, to take advantage of the service does not belong only to the elderly people. Other carers, too, such as Mr Walters' wife, found it unsatisfactory. Mr Walters, aged 97, partially blind, extremely deaf and paralysed down the right side following a stroke, spent two weeks in hospital every eight weeks. His wife, aged 81, and suffering from arthritis, according to the interviewer, did not like him going into hospital but was told he must, periodically, to give her a rest. She visited him daily taking a taxi at £6 a time. Mrs Walters' distress was evident from her remarks.

> They don't care for him as well in hospital as he is cared for at home. He is much more confused than he is when he is at home. Nobody speaks to him and I think he broods and dwells on the past, whereas at home I can talk to him. He gets bored as he can't play his church music or tapes as he does at home. He also has communion two or three times a week at home.
>
> He never comes home without a sore heel or a sore bottom [there was, it seems, also frequent trouble over the emptying of his colostomy bag]. He is supposed to have several drinks a day as he has a catheter, but the cordial I took him some days ago was hardly touched. I took some Bovril in as he doesn't like his meals dry but they refused to put it on.

When Mrs Walters was asked if she needed to talk things over with anyone and how she felt generally about the care she was giving she replied, 'It sounds awful but sometimes I think if I could die I could have a real good rest, but I gabble away to the crucifix for comfort. I don't think he realizes how much I do.' 'But', she continued,

> I wouldn't let him go. I wouldn't be so content for him to live a life like he does just lying in bed. He wouldn't be happy – he was in tears every day in there when he thought he'd got to stop in for good.

During the eight-week periods at home, the district nurse came every day, but Mr Walters was not as satisfied with her as he was with the home help who came on five days a week. Mr Walters, summing up what he felt about respite care, talked of 'being in prison. It's very bad here; there's a shortage of staff and humanity.'

Apart from nursing and home-help services, it might have been expected that when at home Mr Walters and his wife would have had the regular support of their GP. But, despite an apparently good relationship, this was not the case. It had been more than twelve months since the GP's last visit.

General practitioners

In the majority of cases home visits from the general practitioner were more frequent than those to the surgery. The great majority spoke warmly of the relationship they had with their GPs. Mrs Weston described her doctor as a 'friend of the family'. Mr Cleverley put a slightly different point of view. 'It is important that people approach their doctor as a friend and not with fear as most people do – that upsets me. I have found that my way has helped me and I have felt better.'

Generally, there was considerable variation in the regularity with which the elderly people were seen by their GPs, and as many as just over two-thirds said they had no regular contact. Mr Compton, for instance, had 'never had much to do with them. I don't like to bother doctors, they've enough to do without worrying about me.' Furthermore, when asked how long ago they had seen their GP, 15 per cent said that it was more than a year ago. For some, Mr Vincent, for example, the regular weekly or monthly visit was a great support to both carer and cared-for.

149

Screening very old people

We have earlier referred to the WHO categorization of very old people as a 'risk group'. It is, however, recognized by the chief protagonists of the research that has developed the concept of risk groups, that age alone is a doubtful indicator of risk (Taylor 1988). Our evidence corroborates these doubts. It would, nevertheless, be foolish to deny that risks to health increase with age. Regular screening would enable the monitoring of their progress and should be seen in that light, not simply as a means of predicting trouble (Holme and Maizels 1990). Opportunities to set in motion such a procedure would seem generally to be lost in the relatively low involvement of the various professional services. This is not to say that the individuals and their carers are themselves demanding involvement; the evidence from our study suggests otherwise. Any development in screening will therefore have to bridge the gap between professional judgements about need, the apparent lack of interest among many GPs and the personal preference of patients and their families.

Accommodation of the elderly individuals' personal preferences is even more important within an institutional setting, as we suggested in our earlier discussion on dependency and choice. Here, they are extremely vulnerable to the loss of power and the exercise of unwelcome control. The stringent regulations (see e.g. Day and Klein 1987) needed to offset this control are, of course, of a quite different order from those governing the institutions - the workhouse or alms houses – housing elderly people in the days of our sample members' youth, or indeed since that time (see e.g. Townsend 1964). The overtones of the workhouse, if not the actuality, linger on even today.

CARE IN COMMUNAL ESTABLISHMENTS

The care given by the staff of the various establishments in the study consisted mainly of tending activities, though, naturally, this varied according to the type of establishment. A detailed, observational exploration and analysis of this care such as that carried out by Hughes and Wilkin (1987) was beyond the scope of this study. Here, we can only say that 23 per cent of the establishments in the study received some kind of unfavourable comment from the interviewers – severe staff shortages, an inflexible régime, poor atmosphere, little resident/patient autonomy. For a further 10 per cent, the comments were neutral. In none of the former group, however, could signs of abuse or serious neglect be detected, though indifference and some neglect could be inferred, and ungentle attitudes were in evidence.

In ten of the unsatisfactory establishments visited, interviewers specifically criticised relationships between staff and the elderly individuals. They were 'not good', were flawed by a lack of communication or were virtually non-existent – with the obvious risk of neglect – mainly, it seems, because of severe staff shortages. We have had one indication of such neglect in Mr Walters' 'respite' hospital.

Mr Scrutton's interviewer blamed in large part his declared loneliness and boredom on the lack of attention he received, and sympathized with his problems of communication because of 'all these people's southern accent' which he did not understand. A different atmosphere seemed to prevail in Mrs Thrale's nursing home, though the 'laughter and chat' occurred not with her 'carer' but between Mrs Thrale and another nursing assistant. The carer reported this without resentment.

An assessment, which illustrates the tension between subjective perceptions and objective circumstances, was made by the interviewer concerning 99-year-old Mrs Macdonald and her hospital living arrangements. Described as 'a very frail, old lady, cheerful and placid despite severe problems with hearing and sight', she was 'happily settled in a large, long-stay open ward, where she had been for a year'. This was 'cramped and cluttered' with only curtains between the beds. There was a long, narrow, unattractive day/dining room in an old verandah. Mrs Macdonald thought of the staff as 'wonderful' and they were 'obviously attached to her'. The ward sister told the interviewer that there were not enough staff, but they did their best. 'We try to relax routine because it's long stay; patients can make decisions about what time they go to bed and get up.' They also tried to find time to help Mrs Macdonald with dominoes, bingo and draughts which she enjoyed, once she understood what was going on (she refused to wear her hearing aid).

The interviewer of another long-stay patient, described as 'confused, frail, highly dependent and doubly incontinent', referred to the 'understanding and affection' shown by the staff. She nevertheless found it 'tempting to think she might have more personal attention in a private nursing home, though few would accept her'. Her main criticism was of the 'hopeless inaccessibility of the unit for relatives visiting by public transport'.

'Caring attitudes', 'good nursing standards', 'loving and devoted staff' and similar phrases were not infrequently used in the interviewers' assessments. Here, professional commitment had clearly been supplemented by other qualities – 'I love the bones of them all', said one matron. 'It's like having twenty grandmothers', said another. But, just as in a private household setting, the pull of other commitments and duties can undermine relationships. Shortage of staff, pressure of work, whether justifiable or not, were used as 'reasons' by carers, for seemingly casual, or even callous, staff behaviour. Interviewers, and even the elderly people themselves, sometimes agreed. Mrs Short, for instance, found that 'nurses are always saying "Just a moment". One of my fellow residents once replied, "have you any idea how long a moment is?" ' Pressure of work may be so great that 'trivial' requests get forgotten.

SUMMARY

In giving particular weight to the concept of care, especially in the domiciliary setting, rather than of more generalized support, we have seen that the various replies to questions from carers about their role, and from the elderly people about the care they received, involve considerable problems of interpretation. Although we have attempted to link the points of view of both carers and cared-for, relating them to the interviewers' assessments, we still do not always get a complete, or even an adequate picture. A relationship may be fundamentally sound, the devotion real and enduring on either side. This may not be detected in an interview because, at the point – or at some points – of questioning, superficial, recently triggered resentments, hurt feelings or irritations may assume exaggerated, probably temporary, significance. The reverse, of course, is also true. The relationship may have seriously deteriorated but a reluctance to admit this, or to 'complain', or to appear 'uncaring', may result in a misleading impression that all is well.

We have seen that a majority of the informal carers had commitment and the ability to adapt to their situation. They apparently viewed their role with comparative equanimity. An important minority, however, were clearly finding it onerous as far as the restrictions on their own and their family's lives were concerned, and severe – in one or two instances almost unendurable – problems were mentioned by a smaller minority. Sometimes an urgent need to share 'the burden' was expressed, or resentment at the unwillingness of other family members to share it. We have seen also that the majority of the elderly people received the care with appreciation, though a few were, on the face of it, singularly unappreciative, or gave the impression, if not to the interviewer, at least to the carer, of indifference. Perhaps this was justified in ways which we, as researchers, were unable to unravel.

In the residential-care setting, the true state of affairs is even more difficult to establish. On the face of it reasonable, sometimes high, standards of care were apparent in the majority of places. There was no evidence of active ill-treatment or intimidation, though there were, in a small minority of cases, signs of neglect, poor standards of care and ungentle attitudes. A major difference in caring between establishment and private household is that in the former there are likely to be several people involved, compared with only one or two in private households. Because of staff turnover, stability in relationships will suffer, although, paradoxically, if the staff include some who are uncaring, turnover and sheer numbers may be 'protective'. We are, on the whole, persuaded that the many positive assessments of carer/cared-for relationships made by the interviewers, and the appreciative comments by the majority of the establishment residents and patients, had a sound basis.

Looking at more generalized 'support', very old people are regularly in touch with kin and a wider informal network, irrespective of their place of residence, and are, for the most part, firmly supported by them. The professional services play their part and are appreciated, but the extent of their involvement is, perhaps, less than might be expected.

We have in this chapter skirted round the use of the term 'community care' which 'has been talked of for thirty years', and for which 'in few areas can the gap between political rhetoric and policy on the one hand, or between policy and reality in the field on the other hand have been so great' (Griffiths 1988: iv.9). We shall come back to this problem in the next and final chapter.

9

THE ISSUES DISCUSSED

In summarizing the findings of our study of life after 90 we shall seek to show how far we have succeeded in realizing our main aims. These centred on the quality of life, beginning with state of health and material circumstances, including where and with whom the elderly individual was living, and going on to provide a broader view of such issues as leisure activities, questions of 'morale' and well-being (covering feelings of loneliness and boredom), the quality of relationships and the kind of support and care being received. Throughout, we wanted to describe the quality of life in terms of self-reports and self-perceptions. We also wanted to go beyond description, and to explore, where we could, the meanings underlying the relationship between subjective views and objective circumstances.

One of the main purposes of this exercise was to test the proposition that very old age is characterized by diversity, and that differences between men and women, and between those living in private households and those in communal establishments, would be particularly important. At the same time, we expected to find that shared experiences over an exceptionally long life course would produce a common sense of generation, and that this would influence the relationship between social position and outlook on life.

It is perhaps important, at this point, to remind the reader that we set out in the first place to identify and interview a representative sample of individuals aged 90 and over in the belief that, despite the dearth of statistical information and despite warnings that insufficient numbers would be 'interviewable', this was a feasible undertaking. Our belief proved correct. Only 13 per cent of the sample, for instance, needed a proxy for the whole interview. From a methodological point of view, we think we have broken new ground, and we hope that the problems encountered and the procedures followed which are reported in

154

Chapter 1 and Appendix 1 will be useful for future researchers into the subject.

The sample, drawn from eight local authority areas, can claim to be representative of the population of England outside London. Because we were unable to identify the population aged 90 and over in the London borough originally drawn in our stratification procedures, we do not know whether the inclusion of this London borough would have modified our results in any important respect. We believe not.

The proportions of women and men in the sample - four to one – reflected those of the equivalent national population; as did the composition of the two main age groupings 90 – 94 and 95 plus, except that we found a larger proportion of centenarians than we had expected. The oldest member of our sample was aged 106. Roughly equal proportions of the sample were living in private households and in communal establishments, a very different picture from the elderly as a whole. Fewer than 4 per cent, for instance, of those aged 75 to 84 are in residential homes (see Chapter 1).

THE FINDINGS

As we began to analyse the data, diversity among our respondents became apparent, sometimes in the circumstances of the individuals, and sometimes in their evaluations. It also soon became evident that there was a marked sense of generation in the shape of common experiences and attitudes. What emerges is a complex picture of the quality of life after 90.

In some areas the pattern of similiarities and differences can be described with relative clarity. If we look first at objective circumstances, starting with mental and physical health, this is apparent. Throughout the total sample, for example, there was a relatively low prevalence of dementia - 5 per cent - and of serious confusion or memory loss - 14 per cent. In physical health, the great majority reported from one to four chronic conditions, though a small but important minority reported five or more, and a very small group none. There were high levels of sensory impairment among the total sample - no less than 49 per cent and 46 per cent, respectively, with relatively severe or severe deafness and eyesight problems. Arthritis, too, seriously affected nearly half the people in the study. Other long-standing conditions, however, associated with the heart, the lungs or the circulatory system, were less in evidence.

Central to an assessment of health and disability are the questions of mobility and the ability to perform activities of daily living – ADLs – such as washing, dressing, preparing a meal or negotiating stairs. Mobility for the majority was restricted. Nevertheless, a substantial minority of the sample – just over two-fifths – were able to go out, mostly without help; of the housebound majority, again the greater proportion said that they managed on their own without help.

If ADLs, as opposed to mobility, or locomotion, are considered separately, none of these, as might be expected, could be performed by all the members of the sample, even with help. There was, nevertheless, a great range between the sizes of the highest and the lowest proportions saying that they managed easily on their own. Where there were difficulties, many aspects of daily activities shaded into the area of handicap, where the fulfilment of desired roles rather than merely the carrying out of tasks is involved. Such handicap was evident with a minority of the sample members in their inability, for example, to feed themselves, to wash or use the toilet. Larger proportions, but still minorities, were unable, without help, to dress or bath themselves on their own.

As far as the remaining ADLs are concerned, both personal and household, those saying that they could manage easily on their own tended to be smaller minorities than might have been supposed from the proportions saying that they could move around without help. This discrepancy was particularly noticeable in the negotiating of stairs. Here, the picture becomes more complicated, when physical restrictions may be only indirectly related to performing tasks. Changes in motivation and confidence may intervene, creating a difference between the 'can do' and 'do do' aspects of daily life.

The three main components of health and disability – chronic conditions, mobility and ADLs – looked at more closely, varied between those living in private households in the community and those in communal establishments. Significantly higher proportions of individuals belonging to the former group, compared with their counterparts in establishments, were able to carry out such daily tasks. This difference was re-inforced by applying an overall disability measure (percentage disability score (PDS)), which we devised, using the performance ratings of the ADLs. The mean score for those in communal establishments was significantly higher than for those living in private households. The same trend held true for mobility, and also. to an even greater degree, for the relatively few sample members who suffered from incontinence, most of whom were in communal establishments. The causal direction of these findings needs to be treated with care. Whilst it is reasonable to presume that worsening health or disability may precipitate a move from home to a Home, we cannot rule out the possibility that life in a communal establishment may itself generate an increase in difficulties.

Differences in health and disability between men and women were also apparent. Significantly more men had full mobility and a lower level of disability, as measured by the PDS. There were differences, also, in the prevalence of their chronic conditions – more women, proportionately, suffered from arthritis, for example, and had five or more conditions. Another indication of these differences could be seen in the higher proportion of women requiring proxies for the interviews.

As far as material circumstances are concerned, two issues are of particular importance, financial status and the quality of physical surroundings. Unfortunately, our findings on the sample's financial circumstances are limited. Nevertheless, the evidence suggests, with very few but important exceptions, that people aged 90 and over in England are not living in poverty. By the same token, except for a small minority, neither are they living in great affluence; their incomes, as far as we were able to assess them, could be described as adequate. As Jefferys and Thane (1989) have recently pointed out, elderly persons who rely on state pensions and benefits, as two-fifths of our sample members did, are at particular risk from poverty if these are not maintained at an acceptable level. More work certainly needs to be done to reach a fuller understanding of the impact of income and wealth on very old age. The individuals' financial position in communal establishments, for example, is complicated by the presence of minimal personal financial responsibility, and the application of subsidies to meet the costs of both local authority and private residential care.

The social-class position of the sample members is clearly relevant to considerations of past and present financial status. The great majority of the sample belonged to the middle ranks of the class structure, and reported that they had not suffered serious hardship over the life course. Whilst, however, social class remains an influence on material circumstances, we have found that it was of less value in explaining differentials in this sample than were gender and residential status.

For the great majority of our sample members, the physical condition and the standards of amenities in home and Home alike were reasonable and, in some instances, high. There were exceptions – three houses, for example, were without an inside WC, and a few communal establishments were ill-equipped or in poor decorative order. Judgements, however, about the quality of life in relation to material circumstances, as in health, need to take account of subjective responses; and this is even more true when other areas of experience are considered.

In the total sample, for instance, we found a variety of meanings attached to indoor and outdoor leisure pursuits. A few were very active in the sense that they were 'often' engaged in a number of different activities and went out frequently for various purposes – exercise, visits to church, the library, a club (of which they might be the secretary) and so on. Others reported themselves 'busy', too, but they pursued only one or two activities – reading, perhaps, knitting and sewing, or playing bridge. At the other end of the scale, a few had virtually no leisure pursuits, or were not interested in them, usually because of severe physical restrictions. In between were the majority, neither noticeably 'active' nor 'inactive'. Many watched television, listened to the radio or read and, above all, chatted and talked.

In this area, we did not find any marked differences between women and men in the values attached to the various activities. There were, however, differences according to where the sample members were living, but they were not always clear cut. It might be expected, for instance, that chat and talk would occur most frequently in places with 'built-in' company, communal establishments or where the elderly people were living with relatives. In fact, it was those living alone who proportionately mentioned it most often.

Thus, while objective circumstances play an important part in the quality of life in very old age, they do not always operate in a predictable direction. Clearly, good health and material comfort are central components, but they do not necessarily produce a high level of activity, inside or outside the home, and this in turn is not always essential for a good quality of life in the wider sense of well-being.

Our evidence suggests that for the majority of very old people the inevitable acceleration of the ageing process is not accompanied by a sense of frustration and unhappiness. Although, for example, the health of many might be described as poor, it was not, on the whole, evaluated as such by the individuals themselves. Only 8 per cent of the sample members, for instance, rated themselves as unfit or very unfit. This, in very old age, echoes, even more strongly, the general finding that elderly people are inclined to assess their health as good when the 'objective' evidence suggests otherwise (see Chapter 5).

The male/female differences here are worth noting. Although the women had generally a less good state of health than the men, their

158

fitness evaluations did not correspond; the younger women gave a more favourable response than the younger men.

We found a divergence between subjective evaluations of well-being and objective circumstances in several other areas, the former usually presenting a more favourable picture than the latter would seem to warrant. People regularly suffer pain, for example, yet look forward to the day; they are severely restricted physically, yet are never bored; their housing is deficient in amenities such as plumbing, yet it does not, it seems, worry them as they 'have been used to it all [their lives]'; even those few who, by any standards, might be considered poor are reluctant to admit to having to 'go without'.

These kinds of disjunctions were evident among both women's and men's perceptions of their situations, but, with the exception of fitness ratings, women were proportionately more likely than men to find difficulty in coping with daily life and more likely to express negative feelings of well-being; this showed, for example, in the higher prevalence of boredom and loneliness among women (see Chapter 6).

It is, however, important not to exaggerate the effects of subjective evaluations. The presence of other people, for example, seemed to reduce the likelihood of boredom, and the same was true of expressions of loneliness. Under one-fifth of the sample said that they often felt lonely but, where there were such feelings, there was a significant association with the number of hours spent alone.

The availability of company, then, or, more properly, personal relationships, meant much to the great majority of the sample members. Contrary to expectations, there was only a tiny minority who never saw their relatives or had none living. In the support networks children figured prominently, nieces, nephews and other relatives as well; neighbours and friends less so but, where they did, they played a full part. Those living in communal establishments were visited and 'supported' by relatives and, to a limited degree, friends to an extent that confounds the view that once in an 'institution' an old person will be forgotten.

There were naturally differences in the nature of the support received by those living in the two main types of residence. There was more practical help with household chores, for instance, or shopping, given to those in private households. But the extent of 'social and emotional' support was widespread in both settings, and equally valued and appreciated.

Although, as we have discussed in Chapter 8, the problems of interpretation are acute, the majority of the sample expressed satisfaction with the nature and quality of the care they were given, formal and informal. Not everyone, however, in private households was receiving 'care', as distinct from the more generalized, less intimate or demanding 'support' outlined previously, nor indeed, could be said to have been in need of it. But where there were informal carers (in the great majority of cases), nearly all were women, and children predominated. With a few exceptions, the elderly people spoke with gratitude and affection about these informal carers. The affection, accompanied often by emotional ties, was, for the most part, reciprocated. The validity of these positive mutual perceptions was usually corroborated by the interviewers' impressions.

Well over one-third of these daughters, daughters-in-law, nieces and wives devoted the greater part of the day, and sometimes night, to their task. It was clear that, for a minority, the benefits for the elderly people of such care was at considerable cost to the carers. Expressions such as 'physical exhaustion', 'mental strain', even 'desperation' were used. Nevertheless, feelings of resentment were rare though they existed. Within establishments, relationships between carer and cared-for tended to be 'good' but more impersonal, though there were exceptions. Although we found no evidence of abuse or cruelty, there were, in a small minority of establishments, indications of neglect and insensitive behaviour.

We have touched, at various points in our discussion, on the problem of interpreting the underlying meanings of our findings. The fact, for instance, that the majority of individuals reported a relatively 'uneventful' day and at the same time said they were 'never bored', may appear contradictory, but in the context of very old age need not be. Memories of past events and past life, and a sense of achievement over the life course may consciously or unconsciously have provided compensation for inactivity. The absence of positive feelings about the past may help to explain why others in similar circumstances were less happy. On the other hand, generally high levels of satisfaction with such matters as their place of residence, may reflect negative as well as positive features of adaptation, in that being 'institutionalized' may induce an acceptance of what those outside might regard as an unacceptable situation. This raises questions concerning the social context in which choices and preferences are expressed, and the constraints affecting dependency and responsibility, discussed in Chapter 7. For statements of satisfaction may mask the possibility of developing better alternative arrangements, or simply reflect the preferences of other, more powerful, figures in the individual's life.

A part of our original hypothesis, which helps explain these differences, was that the disjuncture between subjective and objective evaluations might have its source in shared generational experiences, through the forming of attitudes arising from historical and biographical events unique to people born at the end of the last century.

This view of the very old as members of a generation, or 'birth cohort', is linked to the outcome of our subsidiary aim – the possible identification of factors that have influenced survival into the tenth decade and beyond – the issue of longevity. As we have discussed in Chapter 3, a survey of very old age cannot provide relevant information on all the factors that have affected the chances of survival amongst the cohort as a whole. Similarly, the factors influencing survival in future cohorts will be very different from those in the present study.

We have, nevertheless, been able to throw some light on relevant biological and social factors. In the first place, of course, are the sex or gender differences evident in the fact (confirmed in our study) that 80 per cent of people aged 90 and over are women. It was also apparent that many of our sample had long-lived parents and, as far as we could discover, long-lived siblings. The recall of the latter was more difficult for most individuals, and the picture for brothers, in particular, is confounded by the high mortality rates during and immediately following the First World War. A substantial minority of people recalled the death of their parents and sisters as being over the age of 80. As we have discussed in Chapter 3, there are difficulties in drawing conclusions about longevity from these findings.

Childhood illness seems to have been largely absent in the lives of our sample members. This may express the impact of social conditions, such as housing and nutrition. In line with this, overall class differences in survival were apparent, as we have mentioned, in favour of middle and upper groups. In combination, sex and class differences produce relatively few male survivors from unskilled manual backgrounds.

Less clear cut, in our evidence, are the associations between survival and life style, except, perhaps concerning smoking. We know that the great majority of males of this cohort as a whole were smokers, many excessive, and many have paid the price in terms of lung and other types of cancers. Few of our own sample members smoked at the time of interview, and, even among the men, most had been life-long moderate or non-smokers. Our evidence on alcohol, and even more so, on diet, is less firm. The association between diet amd survival is currently much in vogue, but few of our sample members conformed to the new rules which have developed in recent years. Diet over the life course had for the majority been remarkable neither for its excesses nor its frugality, nor indeed had it differed much from the habits of the periods they had lived through.

Our sample members, in their subjective perceptions of survival often invoked their way of life, sometimes with overtones of 'moral worth'. From this viewpoint, though only to a limited extent, survival may appear to be a personal achievement or the result of living an 'orderly' and 'proper' life. Few stressed factors such as heredity or social differences.

CONCLUSIONS

We have in this book been exploring 'the paradox of survival'. Living to the age of 90 and over means avoiding or surviving the hazards and trials inevitably encountered in a long life course. Long life also carries the risk of poor health, mental decline and finally, of course, death. While, in one sense, survival may be taken as a sign of being a 'superior' person, in another, the individual runs the ultimate risk of being considered 'inferior', and in turn coming to feel worthless and burdensome.

It is this paradox that helps us understand the positive and negative views about survival into very old age, with which we began the book. Positive views build on a stereotype of the 'superior' survivor and negative views on one of the 'inferior' survivor. As stereotypes they operate in separate compartments – considering them together reveals their contradictory character.

It is true that we have shown some evidence that might be seen to support both these points of view. There are those, as we have seen in the preceding pages, who appear to be 'ageing well', in the sense that they are relatively free from health problems, live in reasonable physical surroundings and are active both inside and outside the home. At the other extreme, we have described individuals with severe difficulties, some of whom were unhappy with life, lonely and frustrated. Others may not even have been interviewed because of dementia or physical decline. But the majority of people over 90 did not fit into either of these categories. Whilst many individuals had 'disengaged' from activities, they remained content, even happy. Social relationships and a sense of fulfilment, or acceptance, often compensated for the losses which time had brought.

The presence of these differences between individuals draws attention to the main conclusion of the study, namely that life after 90 can be compatible with a good quality of life, and is characterized by diversity as well as common problems, or needs. This may have looked different had we studied a wider age group of the very old. We do not know from this study with any certainty whether people aged 90 and over have a better or worse quality of life than those in their 70s or 80s.

The quality of life is marked not only by diversity within the group, but also by complexity in the ageing process for each individual. This partly occurs because of differences in the social circumstances of the very old, whether this arises from differences by virtue of sex, family position or residential status. But it also stems from the many different experiences across a long life course and the historical period over which that life course has unfolded. Modes of upbringing and education, conditions of employment, the First World War, the dramatic social, cultural and economic changes during this century, including changes in the position of women and young people, will all have shaped their responses to present circumstances.

This may in part explain the reluctance we have seen among very old people to complain about their lives, about their financial position, their place of residence or the state of their health. We do not know how later cohorts will react to very old age, but we suspect that they may well show less willingness to accept things as they are, and this is especially true of women, for whom the generational differences in outlook brought about by the feminist movement are considerable. Our findings, for example, on subjective evaluations of fitness may reflect the degree of stoicism involved in the performance of women's customarily imposed gender roles of caring, nurturing, tolerating. How far these generational attitudes will persist in the future is open to question. Similarly, Christian beliefs and the certainty of an after-life were widespread among our sample, and nearness to death seemed to be contemplated, in many instances, with peace of mind. It is difficult to know how far such sources of support and compensation will be turned to by future generations of very old people.

With our study generation, we can say that positive perceptions of earlier achievements and feelings of self-worth may help to compensate for current difficulties. Men, in particular, often look back over a life course marked by activities accorded some degree of public recognition, and this may partly account for the fact that they reported a better sense of life satisfaction, on some measures, than women. Among women, however, there is firm evidence of a widespread serenity of outlook which may derive from close personal relationships, both in the past and in the present.

Our first conclusion on the quality of life in very old age leads us to a second, namely, that realistic national and local planning for the future of very old age is possible, without the sense of gloom that pervades much current debate. There are clearly health and material needs which cannot always be met by the individual or their families. The importance of the need for communal residential care is particularly evident in our study. The postponement, in July 1990, of the NHS Community Care Act reinforces this view. Present government policy, however, seems committed to a reduction in such support.

Similarly, with community care for very old people, despite the fact that recent proposals assign an important *organizing* role to local authorities, there is a danger that the *costs* of caring, both material and emotional, will continue to be carried by individuals and their families. Our study shows that public provision and financial support for the elderly, especially for the very old, will need to remain a priority for the foreseeable future.

The very old, however, are not simply an administrative or medical category, or a new problem group. They do not, on our evidence, threaten to overwhelm the health and welfare services with impossible demands for help. Nor should they run the risk of being blamed for the help they do need. Following Titmuss (1970) and, from a different vantage point, Elias (1985), we suggest that dependence be seen as intrinsic to the lives of everyone, regardless of age or sex, and that reciprocity, either immediate or delayed, is a part of such dependence. Different kinds and degrees of dependency occur at different stages of the life course, and a realistic recognition of its importance in very old age does not mean that it becomes its hallmark.

The needs of very old people, therefore, and this is our third conclusion, should be placed in a context not simply related to age. We hope, on the basis of the empirical evidence of our study, that assessments of 'the oldest old' in the future will be able to draw on and develop the perspectives of the life course and the quality of life in a context which takes account of their past contributions to society, and the present realities of their daily lives.

Finally, we conclude that the improvement in longevity and the growth in numbers of the very old can be regarded as a step forward for society as a whole. The prevention of premature death, and the prolongation of life among older people can therefore be seen as a net gain in human terms.

APPENDIX 1

1 METHOD OF STUDY

In essence the principle of the method of 'probability proportionate to size' (PPS) (Hedges 1977) meant that the larger the proportion of the very old in an area's population the more likely were its chances of selection.

In deciding to use local authority areas for which figures were available on the proportion of the population aged 80 and over, we assumed that the geographical concentration of those over 90 years of age would not differ substantially from those aged 80 and over.

Having obtained the relevant population lists from OPCS, we then divided the total cumulated population by the number of areas required in order to establish a sampling interval, by which we selected the initial twelve areas (see Table A1.1). (For more details on the principles of PPS and an illustrative example, see Hedges 1977: 67.)

2 IDENTIFYING THE 90-PLUS POPULATION

The procedure generally for the statutory services entailed two stages:

First stage

An initial approach to the relevant committee or equivalent responsible body or individual for each area, e.g. for hospital and community-nursing-service patients, the District Medical Ethical Committee(s) (DMEC), for GP patients, the Local Medical Committee (LMC), for social services clients, the Association of Directors of Social Services (ADSS), and for sheltered housing residents, the Director of Housing.

In three areas the health authority and the local authority boundaries

165

Table A.1 The originally selected twelve areas

Interval	Area selection (county)	1983 pop.	% 80+
81,000	Hackney (Greater London)	216,100	2.9
198,630	Wandsworth (Greater London)	258,400	3.4
316,260	Sefton (Merseyside)	299,800	3.4
433,890	Dudley (West Midlands)	300,900	2.4
551,520	Woodspring (Avon)	166,600	3.9
669,150	Carlisle (Cumbria)	101,200	3.4
786,780	Wear Valley (Durham)	88,600	2.3
904,410	New Forest (Hampshire)	149,000	4.4
1,022,040	Maidstone (Kent)	131,300	2.7
1,139,670	Broadland (Norfolk)	98,900	3.0
1,257,300	S Shropshire (Shropshire)	34,200	4.1
1,374,930	Chichester (West Sussex)	99,800	4.4

Source: OPCS 1984, OPCS Monitor

Note: The first sampling unit selected is the one containing the start figure in its range – the sampling interval of 117,630 is then added to 81,000 and so on.

were not co-terminous, which meant that two health authorities for each of these three areas had to be approached.

The applications to the eleven DMECs usually involved completing an elaborate form (a considerable part of which was irrelevant to *social* research), numbers of requests for further clarification and, in one case a personal appearance before the Committee by one of us. The shortest time taken to reach a decision was seven weeks; the longest, seven months. Reasons for the seemingly excessive delays did not all centre on the design and subject matter of the survey. There were also administrative muddles on the part of various committees. All those approached at this stage eventually gave permission for the next stage.

Second stage

Follow-up requests for names, and courtesy letters, to: hospital administrators, consultants, directors of nursing services, etc.; all GPs in the area and FPCs; social services area directors, area officers, research officers, wardens or officers-in-charge of residential homes, etc.; wardens, etc. of sheltered housing units.

As we had discovered when piloting in Wandsworth, passing the first stage did not necessarily mean that those closest to their clients or patients would respond accordingly. For the most part the problem was overcome by the use of consent forms. The solution in Chichester was complex but also successful (see p. 172).

No one type of source – service or agency – was outstandingly better or worse than another, in their willingness to co-operate, in the speed of their response or in the standards of their lists and registers. Within each category, however, there was much variation. Some GPs, directors of nursing services, hospital consultants, housing managers, social services area and research officers, matrons and wardens of homes took endless pains to provide us with the required information, others less so.

Voluntary agencies, private and voluntary homes, churches and the like tended to present fewer obstacles, but on occasions they, too, insisted that prior agreement should be obtained from the elderly individuals for their names to go forward.

3 NATIONAL PROCEDURE FOR NOTIFICATION OF DEATHS

In all cases notification of a death goes from a relative or equivalent person to the district Registrar of Births, Deaths and Marriages and thence to the National Health Services Central Register (NHSCR) at Southport. The Registrar notifies the FPC, who in turn should notify the GP, who should then delete the name from his or her register. Should the patient die at home then notification goes from the GP to the FPC. If the death occurs in hospital, the hospital has an obligation to inform the GP.

4 REVISION OF POPULATION ESTIMATES

The revised population estimates for each area were based on a series of calculations using the original selected sample of 256 by age and sex (see section 5, Table A1.4) and the number of original sample members for whom substitutes had to be found because of pre-identification deaths. The latter were calculated as a percentage of the former and this percentage was then applied to the population age/sex totals for each area.

Where the area population sizes were relatively small, the plus/minus factor would be likely to invalidate any adjustments. For various reasons, it was inadvisable to include Dudley. Table A1.2, therefore, illustrates the results of the calculations for four of the areas.

Table A1.2 Original and revised 90-plus population estimates for four areas

	Chichester	Maidstone	New Forest	Sefton
Women				
90–94				
revised est.	277	291	542	631
original est.	(504)	(291)	(589)	(864)
95+				
revised est.	116	59	135	127
original est.	(247)	(73)	(201)	(270)
Men				
90–94				
revised est.	85	60	92	151
original est.	(146)	(60)	(171)	(186)
95+				
revised est.	32	12	14	18
original est.	(84)	(12)	(54)	(35)
Total				
revised est.	510	422	783	927
original est.	(981)	(436)	(1,015)	(1,355)

5 SELECTION OF THE SAMPLE

The selected sample of 260 was distributed through the eight areas as shown in Table A1.3. To ensure as nationally representative a sample as possible, the 90-plus populations within each of the four age/sex groups in the eight areas were 'pooled' for the purposes of selection. Thereafter, an interval for each sex/age group was calculated.

Table A1.4 shows the reasons why substitutes had to be sought for the out-of-scope sample.

Deaths were discovered of people still registered with GPs, FPCs, social services area offices, which had occurred even as long ago as the 1940s and 50s, and quite often in the 1960s and 70s. The majority of deaths, however, had occurred in the intervening months – or even weeks – since identification. The male 95-plus groups required proportionately the highest number of substitutes.

In table A1.5 we see how the substitute-seeking was distributed through the eight areas.

Table A1.3 Selected sample in the eight areas by sex and age

Areas	Women		Men		Total
	90–94	95+	90–94 (nos)	95+	
Broadland	4	3	6	3	16
Chichester	11	15	10	21	57
Dudley	12	7	9	10	38
Maidstone	5	5	4	3	17
New Forest	11	13	14	13	51
Sefton	16	17	16	8	57
S Shropshire	3	3	3	2	11
Wear Valley	3	1	3	2	9
Total	65	64	65	62	256[a]

[a] Four individuals were 'lost' to the selected number of 260 because of mis-information coming too late to rectify.

Table A1.4 Reasons for non-availability of the out-of-scope individuals drawn in the initial sampling

Reasons	Subjects nos
Dead	447
Untraceable/presumed dead	60
Moved out of area	15
Wrong date of birth/information	17
Total	539

The excessive number of substitutes in Chichester was due partly to the fact that the original trawl among the various services and agencies (except for social services) occurred during the pilot phase a year earlier than in the other areas, and partly to a failure on the part of the social services department to update their records – a failure in which they were by no means alone.

6 METHOD OF WEIGHTING

In order to arrive at the appropriate weight for each of the four age/sex groups a series of calculations was made, based on national

Table A1.5 Subjects in the eight areas for whom one or more substitutes were selected

Study areas	Selected sample	No. of substitutes			
		One	Two	Three or more	Total no. of subjects needing substitutes
				Nos	
Broadland	16	2	1	–	3
Chichester	57	42	36	292	370
Dudley	38	13	7	9	29
Maidstone	17	6	4	2	12
New Forest	51	23	10	9	42
Sefton	57	22	9	6	37
S Shropshire	11	1	1	2	4
Wear Valley	9	4	3	4	11
Total	256	113	71	324	508

Table A1.6 Sample composition by sex and age: actual and weighted numbers

		Actual sample	Weighted sample	
Women	90–94	46	x 2.7	124
	95+	47	x 0.77	36
	total	133		160
Men	90–94	54	x 0.63	34
	95+	36	x 0.17	6
	total	90		40
Total subjects		183		200

population estimates and our interviewed sample numbers (see Table A1.6).

7 CENTENARIANS

The difficulty of identifying *living* people aged 90 and over worsens the older they become and for centenarians there is an admission of this problem among the compilers of national statistics (Thatcher 1981: 11–14). Sifting the evidence from 1981 Census and DHSS returns at a later date, the Registrar General estimated that the most reliable estimate of centenarian numbers for 1981 was 2,410 (OPCS 1985: 13). In the 1981 census the figure for people aged 90 and over was estimated at 146,423 (OPCS 1983: 6). Centenarians would therefore have constituted 1.6 per cent of the 1981 90-plus population.

Since, however, the official 90-plus estimates are admitted to be less reliable than those for younger ages, there must be some doubt on estimates of centenarians. Our considerably higher proportion of 7.7 per cent (222/17), therefore, should be seen in this light. It may be that the omission of a London borough is responsible for the higher proportions in our study.

8 MAIN AREAS OF QUESTIONING

The main questionnaire was divided into four main sections. The first – THE PAST – dealt with personal history, including places of birth and upbringing, previous residence, education, employment, health, key events throughout life and familial history – particularly the age at death of parents and siblings. Questions also covered present residence, and preferences and reasons for being there.

The longest section – THE PRESENT – focused primarily on the quality of life, on their regular daily activities, leisure, mobility, physical and mental-health status (including respondents' own views on this), on related issues (medicines, sleep patterns, smoking, alcohol consumption, diet, etc.), the extent of informal and formal support and how it was valued and on financial circumstances. It also contained questions on morale and attitudes – loneliness, boredom, worries, feelings about old age and so on. The third section – INFORMATION – asked for household particulars, housing type and tenure, type of institution, amenities, etc. Finally, the INTERVIEWER'S ASSESS-MENT contained twelve questions, some precoded, some open-ended, concerning the interview, the interviewee, the quality of the relationship between subject and carer, the residence and living arrangements.

9 THE MAIN SOURCES CONSULTED FOR QUESTIONNAIRE DESIGN

For general survey methods on the elderly:

Questionnaire of the study in North Wales of elderly people in the community (Wenger 1984).

Interview schedule of a survey of elderly people in Sheffield, 1985, Dept of Sociological Studies, University of Sheffield.

For physical and mental health measures and assessments concerning the elderly:

Physical and psychological schedule used for a Research Project on Services for the Elderly, 1985, University Hospital of South Manchester.

Questionnaire used for the Nottingham Health Profile (Hunt *et al.* 1980).

The modified Crichton Royal Behavioural Rating Scale (Goldberg and Connelly, 1983).

Questionnaire used for the Aberdeen study on ageing (Taylor *et al.* 1983).

Interview schedule used for the Geriatric Mental State (GMS) Study 1985, Department of Psychiatry, Royal Liverpool Hospital.

10   METHOD OF APPROACH TO RESPONDENTS

Letters briefly explaining the project and asking for an interview were prepared for each selected subject and sent, with a covering letter to the person from whom we had received the subject's name for signature and despatch. A courtesy letter was sent to any secondary sources. No-one failed to undertake this on our behalf.

The problem of anonymity for the Chichester Social Services list was overcome as follows: The same member of the department who had originally compiled their list and compared it with ours carried out the interviews of anyone on their lists, following the same procedures as the other interviewers.

11   DATA ANALYSIS

(a) The SPSSx package. Since no previous study of a representative sample of people aged 90 and over had ascertained the extent of their ability to give meaningful answers, we decided to concentrate on providing a general, but as far as possible, precise picture of the life course and daily life of the respondents.

To analyse the quantifiable data we employed the computer statistical package, SPSSx. Where appropriate, we developed measures (for example, scaling disability items) and established associations which could be exposed to tests of significance. Statistically significant results have been referred to as such in the text by the word 'significant' where appropriate. In the main, however, we have used the data to describe and to generate ideas rather than concentrate on statistical associations, let alone causal relationships between phenomena.

(b) Since a number of the sample members were very frail, or had difficulty because of deafness, dementia and the like, in communicating continuously, there was variation in the total numbers replying to each question. Where tables are used the totals are shown; where proportions are referred to only in the text, the reader may assume that these are based on a size not smaller than two-thirds of the appropriate sample size unless otherwise stated.

(c) Following Wenger's (1988: 4) practice, generalized terms are sometimes used to indicate proportions. In our case the following are those mainly used:

the great majority/most	= more than three-quarters
the majority/many	= over one-half – three-quarters
some/a minority	= one-quarter – under one-half
a small minority/a few	= under one-quarter

(d) The data have been analysed for the 90-plus population of the eight areas taken as a whole rather than by area. Our main aim was to study a nationally representative sample in order to overcome criticisms that can be laid against findings drawn from a single geographical location, particularly as the area numbers in this case were relatively small.

APPENDIX 2

SUPPLEMENTARY TABLES

Tables referred to in chapters 2, 3, 4, 6 and 8

Table A2.1 Age of leaving school by sex: weighted sample

Age	Women %	Men %
12 and under	9.2	10.3
13	18.3	17.9
14	47.9	43.6
15/16	6.3 } 24.6	17.9 } 28.2
17/18	18.3	10.3
Total	100	100
	(142)	(39)

Table A2.2 Residence in private households and communal establishments by sex and age: actual sample

Type of residence	Women		Men	
	90–94	95+	90–94	95+
		Nos		
Private households	23	15	32	19
Communal establishments	23	32	22	17
Total	46	47	54	36

174

Table A2.3 Age at death of sisters (numbering one to five only) by sex: weighted sample

Age at death of sisters	Women %	Men %
39 and under	11.7	12.5
40–59	7.8	12.5
60–69	10.0	5.0
70–79	31.7	32.5
80+	38.7	37.5
Total no. of sisters	100[1]	100
	(230)	(40)
Total no. of subjects	(99)	(20)

[1]See note 2.

Table A2.4 Age at death of brothers (numbering one to five only) by sex: weighted sample

Age at death of brothers	Women %	Men %
39 and under	19.3	28.6
40–59	15.5	13.8
60–69	19.3	17.2
70–79	17.6	25.9
80+	28.3	15.5
Total no. of brothers	100	100
	(233)	(58)
Total no. of subjects	(105)	(26)

Table A2.5 Social-class comparisons between sample members and their fathers: weighted sample

Social class		Fathers %	Sample members %
I	Professional, etc.	10.2	15.7
II	Intermediate	25.0	21.3
III.1	Skilled non-manual	5.1	9.6
III.2	Skilled manual	40.3	36.0
IV	Partly skilled	14.2	11.8
V	Unskilled	5.1	5.6
		100[1]	100
Total subjects		(176)	(187)

[1]See note 2.

Table A2.6 Drinking habits by sex in England and Wales 1984

Type of drinker	Males %	Females %
Abstainer	7	13
Occasional	9	20
Infrequent light	12	19
Frequent light	38	42
Moderate	14	4
Heavy	20	2

Source: CSO 1988

Table A2.7 Frequency of intake of different foodstuffs: weighted sample

Type of foodstuff	Rare %	Occas. %	At least weekly %	Daily %	Total subjects n=190 %
Meat	2.2	4.0	13.0	80.8	100
Fish	4.4	17.6	74.0	3.9	100[1]
Poultry	3.6	18.3	68.6	9.4	100[1]
Fresh milk	4.8	5.4	5.9	83.9	100
Eggs	15.5	20.4	44.9	19.1	100[1]
Fresh fruit	9.7	13.7	24.0	52.6	100
Fresh vegetables	1.0	8.1	6.8	84.0	100[1]
Wholemeal bread	34.7	11.7	8.1	45.5	100

[1]See note 2.

Table A2.8 Number of reported chronic conditions per person: weighted sample

No. of conditions per person	%
0	7.2
1	15.0
2	29.3
3 or 4	34.1
5 or more	14.4
Total subjects	100
	(200)

Table A2.9 Prevalence of pain by sex and age: actual sample

	Women		Men	
	90–94	95+	90–94	95+
		Nos		
No	12	27	25	16
Yes	30	18	25	20
Total subjects	42	45	50	36

Table A2.10 Frequency of urinary incontinence by type of residence: weighted sample

Frequency	Private households %	Communal establishments %
Never	91.1	68.2
Twice a week or less	2.1	5.0
Three–six times a week	0.8	0.8
Daily or more	5.9	25.9
Total subjects	100[1]	100
	(92)	(95)

[1]See note 2.

Table A2.11 Frequency of bowel incontinence by type of residence: weighted sample

Frequency	Private households %	Communal establishments %
Never	91.2	77.8
Twice a week or less	6.0	9.2
Three–six times a week	2.8	5.1
Daily or more	0.0	7.9
Total subjects	100	100
	(96)	(95)

Table A2.12 Comparison of activities of daily living in private households and communal establishments: weighted sample

	Can do easily or alone with difficulty	
	Private household % n=94	Communal establishments % n=96
Feeding yourself	92	48
Washing (face and hands)	91	66
Using toilet	89	61
Dressing	81	19
Combing hair/shaving	80	67
Preparing a meal	73	–
Light domestic jobs	62	–
Negotiating steps	55	32
Bathing	53	22
Fiddly jobs like sewing on buttons	47	27
Negotiating stairs	46	26
Writing letters to family and friends	44	29
Cutting toenails	35	14

APPENDIX 2

Table A2.13 Frequency of contact with relatives (excepting spouse and individuals living with relatives) by type of residence: weighted sample

Frequency of contact	Living in:	
	Private households %	Communal establishments %
Never	2.1	4.5
Less than monthly	18.0	10.7
At least once a month	3.1	21.6
At least once a week	34.4	42.4
(Almost) daily	42.4	20.8
Total	100	100
	(66)	(98)

NOTES

1 In 1961 the standardized mortality ratio (SMR) for coal-face miners aged from 15–64 was 180; that of university teachers, fifty-six (Tuckett 1976).
2 The percentages do not add up to 100, due to the re-weighting of the sample numbers.
3 The differences between the actual sample numbers (94) living in communal establishments and the numbers of establishments (86) is accounted for by the fact that: two individuals were in the same long-stay hospital; two were in the same local authority home; two were in one private residential home and two in another.
4 We considered ways in which we could arrive at an overall disability score, but because of our sample characteristics this became too complicated to put into operation. In particular the weights attached to individual items would have had to take into account the very different circumstances of our sample members – the differences, for instance, between residence in private households and communal establishments. Our more simple PDS did enable us to make meaningful distinctions between individuals and groups.

REFERENCES

Abercrombie, N., Warde, A., Soothill, K., Urry, J. and Walby, S. (1988) *Contemporary British Society*, Oxford: Basil Blackwell.

Abrams, M. (1978) *Beyond Three Score and Ten (A first report on a survey of the elderly)*, Mitcham: Age Concern.

Abrams, M. (1988) 'The elderly today 2: a social audit', in N. Wells and C. Freer (eds) *The Ageing Population*, London: Macmillan.

Abrams, P. (1984) 'Realities of neighbourhood care', in M. Bulmer, (ed.) *Policy and Politics*, 12 (4), 413–429.

Age Concern (1974) *The Attitudes of the Retired and Elderly*, Mitcham: Age Concern.

Age Concern (1978) *Profiles of the Elderly 4*, Mitcham: Age Concern.

Allan, G. (1979) *A Sociology of Friendship and Kinship*, London: Allen & Unwin.

Anderson, M. (1971) *Family Structure in Nineteenth-Century Lancashire*, Cambridge: Cambridge University Press.

Anderson, R. (1987) 'The unremitting burden of carers', *British Medical Journal*, 294, 73–4.

Anderson, R. (1988) 'The quality of life of stroke patients and their "carers" ', in R. Anderson and M. Bury (eds) (see Anderson and Bury (1988)).

Anderson, R. and Bury, M. (eds) (1988) 'Introduction', *Living with Chronic Illness, The Experience of Patients and Their Families*, London: Unwin Hyman.

Andrews, B. and Brown, G. W. (1988) 'Social support, onset of depression and personality: an exploratory analysis', *Social Psychiatry & Psychiatric Epidemiology*, 23, 99–108.

Arber, S. and Gilbert, N. (1989) 'Men: the forgotten carers', *Sociology*, 23 (1), 111–18.

Armstrong, D. (1983) *Political Anatomy of the Body, Medical Knowledge in Britain in the 20th Century*, Cambridge: Cambridge University Press.

Attenburrow, J. (1976) *Grouped Housing for the Elderly*, DOE, England: Building Research Establishment.

Barker, J. and Bury, M. R. (1978) 'Mobility and the elderly: a community challenge', in V. Carver and P. Liddiard (eds) *An Ageing Population*, Sevenoaks: Hodder & Stoughton (in association with Open University Press, Milton Keynes).

Baylis, R., Clarke, C. and Whitfield, G. (1986) 'The female life span', *Journal of the Royal College of Physicians,* 20 (4), 290–3.

Blaxter, M. (1976) *The Meaning of Disability,* London: Heinemann.

Blythe, R. (1969) *Akenfield, Portrait of an English Village,* Harmondsworth: Penguin.

Bond, J. (1987) 'Health Policy (Abstracts)', *Ageing and Society,* 7 (4), 473–6, Cambridge: Cambridge University Press.

Booth, T. (1985) *Home Truths: Old People's Homes and the Outcome of Care,* Aldershot: Gower.

Booth, T. (1986) 'Institutional régimes and residential outcomes in homes for the elderly', in C. Phillipson, M. Bernard and P. Strang (eds) *Dependency and Interdependence in Old Age,* London: Croom Helm.

Bowling, A., Hart, D. and Silman, A. (1989) 'Accuracy of electoral registers and family practitioner committee lists for population studies of the very elderly', *Journal of Epidemiology and Community Health,* 43, 391–394.

Bowling, A., Hoeckel, T. and Leaver, J. (1988) *Health and Social Service Needs for People Aged 85 and Over Living in City and Hackney,* London: Dept. of Community Medicine, City and Hackney Health Authority.

Brearley, C. P. (1982) *Risk and Ageing,* London: Routledge & Kegan Paul.

Bredemeier, H. C. (1978) 'Exchange theory', in T. Bottomore and R. Nisbet (eds), *A History of Sociological Analysis,* London: Heinemann.

Brody, J. A. (1985) 'Prospects for an ageing population', *Nature,* 315, 463–6.

Brown, G. W. and Harris, T. (1978) *The Social Origins of Depression,* London: Tavistock.

Buchanan, J. M. and Chamberlain, M. A. (1978) *Survey of the Mobility of the Disabled in an Urban Environment,* London: The Royal Association for Disability and Rehabilitation.

Bucke, M. and Insley, M. L. (1976) 'Centenarians are healthy, but they need mental and emotional care', *Modern Geriatrics,* 6 (2), 24–8

Bulmer, M. (1987) *The Social Basis of Community Care,* London: Allen & Unwin.

Bury, M. R. (1982) 'Chronic illness as biographical disruption', *Sociology of Health and Illness,* 4 (2), 167–82.

Bury, M. R. (1986) 'Social constructionism and the development of medical sociology, *Sociology of Health and Illness,* 8 (2), 137–69.

Bury, M. (1988) 'Arguments about ageing: long life and its consequences', in N. Wells and C. Freer (eds) *The Ageing Population,* London: Macmillan.

Butler, A., Oldman, C. and Greve, J. (1983) *Sheltered Housing for the Elderly: Policy, Practice and the Consumer,* London: Allen & Unwin.

Calnan, M. (1987) *Health and Illness: The Lay Perspective,* London: Tavistock.

Carley, M. (1981) *Social Measures and Social Indicators: issues of policy and theory,* London: Allen & Unwin.

Cartwright, A., Hockey, L. and Anderson, J. C. (1973) *Life Before Death,* London: Routledge & Kegan Paul.

Cassileth, B. R., Lusk, E. J., Strouse, T. B. *et al.* (1984) Psychosocial status in chronic illness: a comparative analysis of six diagnostic groups', *New England Journal of Medicine* 311, 506–10.

Challis, L. and Bartlett, H. (1988) *Old and Ill, Private Nursing Homes for Elderly People,* Inst. of Gerontology, Research Paper 1, Mitcham: Age Concern.

Challis, D. and Davies, B. (1988) 'The community care approach: an innovation in home care by social services department', in N. Wells and C. Freer (eds) *The Ageing Population*, London: Macmillan.

Clarke, C. (1986) 'Increased longevity in man', *Journal of the Royal College of Physicians*, 20 (2), 122.

Clarke, C. (1987) Personal communication.

Cm 849 (1989) *Caring for People: Community Care in the Next Decade and Beyond*, DSS White Paper, London: HMSO.

Cochrane, A. (1972) *Effectiveness and Efficiency in The National Health Service*, Oxford: Nuffield Provincial Hospital Trust.

Crawford, R. (1977) 'You are dangerous to your health: the ideology and politics of victim blaming', *International Journal of Health Services*, 7, 663–80.

CSO (1955) *Annual Abstract of Statistics*, 92, London: HMSO.

CSO (1988) *Social Trends*, 18, London: HMSO.

CSO (1989a) *Social Trends*, 19, London: HMSO.

CSO (1989b) *Annual Abstract of Statistics*, London: HMSO.

Day, P. and Klein, R. (1987) 'Quality of institutional care and the elderly: policy issues and options', *British Medical Journal*, 294, 384–7.

DOE (1977) *Housing Policy, Tech Vol*, Part 1, London: HMSO.

Dubos, R. (1960) *Mirage of Health*, London: Allen & Unwin.

Elias, N. (1985) *The Loneliness of Dying*, Oxford: Basil Blackwell.

Evandrou, M., Arber, S., Dale, A. and Gilbert, G. N. (1986) 'Who cares for the elderly? Family care provision and receipt of statutory services', in C. Phillipson, H. Bernard and P. Strang (eds) *Dependency and Interdependence in Old Age*, London: Croom Helm.

Evans, G. J. (1983) 'The appraisal of hospital geriatric services', *Community Medicine*, 3, 242–50.

Falkingham, J. (1987) 'Britain's ageing population: the engine behind increased dependency?' *The Welfare State Programme*, Discussion Paper 17, London: London School of Economics.

Fallo-Mitchell, L. and Ryff, C. D. (1982) 'Preferred timing of female life events; cohort differences', *Research on Aging*, 4 (2), 249–67.

Fennell, G., Phillipson, C. and Evers, H. (1988) *The Sociology of Old Age*, Milton Keynes: Open University Press.

Ferguson, S. (1975) *Drink*, London: B. T. Batsford Ltd.

Finch, J. and Groves, D. (1983) (eds) *A Labour of Love: Women, Work and Caring*, London: Routledge & Kegan Paul.

Ford, G. and Taylor, R. (1985) 'The elderly as underconsulters: a critical reappraisal', *Journal of the Royal College of General Practitioners*, 35, 244.

Fox, A. J., Goldblatt, P. O. and Jones, D. R. (1985) 'Social class morality differentials: artefact selection or life circumstances?' *Journal of Epidemiology and Community Medicine*, 39, 1.

Freer, C. (1988) 'Old myths; frequent misconceptions about the elderly', in N. Wells and C. Freer (eds) *The Ageing Population*, London: Macmillan.

Freidson, E. (1970) *Profession of Medicine*, New York: Dodd Mead.

Fries, J. F. (1980) 'Aging, natural death and the compression of morbidity', *New England Journal of Medicine*, 3 (50), 303.

George, L. K. and Bearon, L. B. (1980) *Quality of Life in Older Persons: Meaning and Measurement*, New York: Human Science Press.

Glendenning, C. and Millar, J. (eds) (1987) *Women and Poverty in Britain*, Brighton: Wheatsheaf.

Goldberg, E. M. and Connelly, N. (1983) *The Effectiveness of Social Care for the Elderly*, London: Heinemann.

Gordon, C. (1989) 'Familial support for the elderly in the past: the case of London's working class in the early 1930s', *Ageing and Society*, 8 (2), Cambridge: Cambridge University Press.

Gouldner, A. W. (1960) 'The norm of reciprocity: a preliminary statement', *American Sociological Review*, 25 (2), 162–78.

Gove, W. (1973) 'Sex, marital status and mortality', *American Journal of Sociology*, 79, 45–67.

Gray, J. A. M. (1988) 'Living environments for the elderly', in N. Wells and C. Freer (eds) *The Ageing Population*, London: Macmillan.

Griffiths, R. (1988) (Chairman) *Community Care: Agenda for Action*, A Report to the Secretary of State for Social Services, London: HMSO.

Halsey, A. H. (1986) *Change in British Society*, 3rd edn, Oxford: Oxford University Press.

Harman, H. and Harman, S. (1989) *No Place Like Home*, A Report of the First Ninety-Six Cases of the Registered Homes Tribunal, NALGO.

Havighurst, R. J. (1951) 'Validity of the Chicago Adjustment Inventory as a measure of personal adjustment in old age', *Journal of Abnormal and Social Psychology*, 46, 24–9.

Hedges, B. (1977) 'Sampling', in Hoinville, G. and Jowell, R. (eds) *Survey Research Practice*, London: Heinemann.

Hicks, C. (1988) *Who Cares: Looking after People at Home*, London: Virago.

Holme, A. (1985) *Housing and Young Families in East London*, London: Routledge & Kegan Paul.

Holme, A. and Maizels, J. (1990) 'Seventy plus, a study of the health care needs of older people in Brent, for Age Concern, Brent', in M. Bury and J. Macnicol (eds) *Aspects of Ageing*, Social Policy Papers 3, Dept. of Social Policy and Social Science, RHBNC.

Horley, J. (1984) 'Life satisfaction, happiness and morale: two problems with the use of the subjective well-being indicators', *The Gerontologist*, 24, 2.

Hughes, B. and Wilkin, D. (1987) 'Physical care and quality of life in residential homes', *Ageing and Society*, 7 (4) 399–425, Cambridge: Cambridge University Press.

Hunt, A. (1978) *The Elderly at Home*, OPCS, Social Survey Division, London: HMSO.

Hunt, S. M., McKenna, S. P., McEwen, J., Backett, E. M., Williams, J. and Papp, E. (1980) 'A quantitative approach to perceived health status: a validation study', *Journal of Epidemiology and Community Health*, 34 (4), 281–86.

Ignatieff, M. (1984) *The Needs of Strangers*, London: Hogarth Press.

Illsley, R. (1980) *Professional or Public Health,* Oxford: Nuffield Provincial Hospital Trust.

Jefferys, M. and Thane, P. (1989) 'An ageing society & ageing people', in Jefferys, M. (ed.) *Growing Old in the Twentieth Century*, London: Routledge.

Jefferys, M. (1990) 'The elderly in society', in J. C. Brocklehurst, R. C. Tallis and H. Fillit (eds) *Textbook of Geriatric Medicine and Gerontology* (4th edn), London: Churchill Livingstone.

Johnson, M. L. (1984) 'Privatising residential care: a review of changing policy and practice', in Laming, H. (ed.) *Residential Care for the Elderly*, London: Policy Studies Institute.

Jones, D. A. and Vetter, N. J. (1984) 'A survey of those who care for the elderly at home: their problems and their needs', *Social Science & Medicine,* 19 (5), 511–14.

Kalache, A., Warnes, T. and Hunter, D. J. (1988) *Promoting Health Among Elderly People,* London: King Edward's Hospital Fund for London.

Kholi, M. (1988) 'Ageing as a challenge to sociological theory', *Ageing and Society* 8 (4), 367–94, Cambridge: Cambridge University Press.

Knapp, R. J. (1977) 'The activity theory of aging: an examination in the English context', *The Gerontologist,* 17 (6), 553.

Laing, W. (1988) 'Living environments for the elderly, 3, the mixed economy in long-term care', in N. Wells and C. Freer (eds) *The Ageing Population,* London: Macmillan.

Land, H. (1978) 'Who Cares for the Family?' *Journal of Social Policy,* 7 (3), 357–84.

Land, H. (in press) 'The changing boundaries of community care', in J. Gabe, M. Calnan and M. Bury (eds) *The Sociology of the Health Service,* London: Routledge.

Laslett, P. (1972) *The World We have Lost* (2nd edn), London: Methuen.

Laslett, P. (1987) 'The emergence of the third age', *Ageing and Society,* 7 (2), 133–60, Cambridge: Cambridge University Press.

Laslett, P. (1989) *A Fresh Map of Life: The Emergence of the Third Age,* London: Weidenfeld & Nicolson.

Levkoff, S. E., Cleary, P. D. and Wetle, T. (1986) 'Differences in the appraisal of health between aged and middle-aged adults', *Journal of Gerontology,* 42, 114–120.

Loomes, G. and McKenzie, L. (1988) 'Use of QALYS in health care decision making', *Social Science and Medicine* 28 (4), 289–308.

MacIntyre, S. (1986) 'The patterning of health by social position in contemporary Britain, directions for sociological research', *Social Science & Medicine,* 22 (4), 393–415.

Macnicol, J. (1990) 'The concept of "structured dependency" ', in M. Bury and J. Macnicol (eds) *Aspects of Ageing,* Social Policy Papers 3, Dept. of Social Policy and Social Science, RHBNC.

Marmot, M., Kogevinas, M. and Elston, M. A. (1987) 'Social/economic status and disease', *Annual Review of Public Health,* 8, 111–35.

Marmot, M., Rose, G., Shipley, M. and Hamilton, P. J. S. (1978) 'Employment grade and coronary heart disease in British civil servants', *Journal of Epidemiology and Community Health,* 32, 244–9.

Martin, J., Meltzer, H. and Elliot, D. (1988) *The Prevalence of Disability Among Adults,* OPCS Surveys of Disability in Gt. Britain, Report No. 1, London: HMSO.

Maynard, A. (1989) 'Creating an efficient market for care of the elderly', *Generation,* 9, 47–58, BSG Bulletin.

Mechanic, D. (1968) *Medical Sociology,* New York: Free Press.

Medley, M. L. (1980) 'Life satisfactions across four stages of adult life', *International Journal of Aging and Human Development* 11.

Middleton, L. (1987) *So Much for So Few: A View of Sheltered Housing,* Liverpool: The Institute of Human Ageing, Liverpool University Press.

Millard, P. (1985) Personal communication.

MMF (Millbank Memorial Fund) *Quarterly* (1985).

Morton-Williams, J. (1979) *Alternative Patterns of Care for the Elderly* (Methodological report for a study designed by the Institute for Economic and Social Research, University of York), London: Social and Community Planning Research.

Murphy, E. (1982) 'The social origins of depression in old age', *British Journal of Psychiatry*, 141, 135–42.

Mutran, E. and Reitzes, D. C. (1981) 'Retirement, identity and well-being: realignment of role relationships', *Journal of Gerontology*, 36 (6), 733–40.

Najman, J. M. and Levine, S. (1981) 'Evaluating the impact of medical care and technologies on the quality of life: a review and critique', *Social Science & Medicine*, 15 (2), 102–16.

Nathanson, C. (1975) 'Illness and the feminine role: a theoretical review', *Social Science & Medicine*, 9, 57–62.

Norman, A. (1980) *Rights and Risks*, NCCOP, London: Centre for Policy on Ageing.

O'Connor, D. W., Pollitt, P. A., Brook, C. P. B. and Reiss, B. B. (1989) (in press) 'A community survey of mental and physical infirmity in nonagenarians', *Age and Ageing*.

OPCS (1977) *GHS*, 7, London: HMSO.

OPCS (1983a) *Census 1981 National Report GB Part 1*, London: HMSO.

OPCS (1983b) *Census 1981 National Report, General Notes: Communal Establishments*, London: HMSO.

OPCS (1984) Census 1981, *The Proportion of Elderly People in each Local Authority District of Great Britain, 1981*, Key statistics for local authorities, London: HMSO.

OPCS (1985a) *Population Projections*, series PP2: 13, London: HMSO.

OPCS (1985b) *Population Trends 40*, London: HMSO.

OPCS (1989) *GHS* 16, 1986, London: HMSO.

Oppenheim, A. N. (1966) *Questionnaire Design and Attitude Measurement*, London: Heinemann.

Parker, R. (1981) 'Tending and social policy', in E. M. Goldberg and S. Hatch (eds) *A New Look at the Personal Social Services*, Discussion Paper No. 4, London: Policy Studies Institute.

Parsons, T. (1951) *The Social System*, London: Routledge & Kegan Paul.

Patrick, D. (1986) 'Measurement of health and quality of life', in D. L. Patrick and G. Scambler (eds) (2nd edn) *Sociology As Applied to Medicine*, London: Baillier & Tindall.

Peace, S. (1988) 'Living environment for the elderly. Promoting the "right" institutional environment', in N. Wells and C. Freer (eds) *The Ageing Population*, London: Macmillan.

Pooley, L. (1988) 'Havens or ghettos for the elderly?' *Independent*, 19 Oct 88.

Powles, J. (1978) 'The effect of health services on adult male mortality in relation to the effect of social and economic factors', *Ethics, Science and Medicine*, 5 (1).

Ragheb, M. G. and Griffiths, C. A. (1982) 'The contribution of leisure participation and leisure satisfaction of older persons', *Journal of Leisure Research*, 14 (4), 295–306.

Rastan, C. (1989) 'Angels who are more than guardians', *The Independent*, 20 June 1989.

Ridley, J. C., Bachrach, C. A. and Dawson, D. A. (1979) 'Recall and reliability of interview data from older women', *Journal of Gerontology*, 34 (1).

Riley, M. W., Phoner, A. and Waring, J. (1988) 'The sociology of age', in N. J. Smelser (ed.) *Handbook of Sociology*, London: Sage.

Roberts, R. (1973) *The Classic Slum*, Harmondsworth: Penguin.

Rowntree, B. S. (1901) *A Study of Town Life*, London: Macmillan.

Shanas, E., Townsend, P., Wedderburn, D., Hemming, F., Milhof, P. and Stehouwer, J. (1968) *Old People in Three Industrial Societies*, London: Routledge & Kegan Paul.

Sinclair, I., Crosbie, D., O'Connor, P., Stanforth, L. and Vickey, A. (1984) *A Study of Informal Care, Services and Social Work for Elderly Clients Living Alone*, London: National Institute for Social Work Research Unit.

Spark, M. (1959) *Momento Mori*, London: Macmillan.

Staats, S. R. and Stasson, M. A. (1987) 'Age and present and future perceived quality of life', *International Journal of Aging and Human Development*, 25 (3), 167–76.

Stimson, G. V. C. (1974) 'Obeying doctor's orders: a view from the other side', *Social Science & Medicine*, 8, 97–105.

Stones, M. J. and Kozma, A. (1986) 'Happiness and activities as propensities', *J. of Gerontology*, 41 (1), 85–90.

Strauss, A. (1975) *Chronic Illness and the Quality of Life*, St Louis: Mosby.

Taylor, L. and Mullan, R. G. (1986) *Uninvited Guests, The Intimate Secrets of Television and Radio*, London: Chatto & Windus.

Taylor, R. (1988) 'The elderly as members of society: an examination of social differences in an elderly population', in N. Wells and C. Freer (eds) *The Ageing Population*, London: Macmillan.

Taylor, R., Ford, G. and Barber, H. (1983) *The Elderly at Risk: Research Perspectives on Ageing*, Mitcham: Age Concern Research Unit.

Thatcher, A. R. (1981) 'Centenarians', *Population Trends*, 25, 11.

Tinker, A. (1984) *The Elderly in Modern Society*, 2nd edn, London: Longman.

Titmuss, R. (1970) *The Gift Relationship*, London: Allen & Unwin.

Topliss, E. (1975) *Provision for the Disabled*, Oxford: Basil Blackwell.

Townsend, P. (1957) *The Family Life of Old People*, London: Routledge & Kegan Paul.

Townsend, P. (1964) *The Last Refuge,* London: Routledge & Kegan Paul.

Townsend, P. (1979) *Poverty in the United Kingdom,* Harmondsworth: Penguin.

Townsend, P. (1981) 'The structured dependency of the elderly: a creation of social policy in the twentieth century', *Ageing and Society*, 1 (1), 5–28, Cambridge: Cambridge University Press.

Townsend, P. (1989) 'The social & economic hardship of elderly people in London', *Generations* 9, 10–129, BSG.

Townsend, P., Davidson, N. and Whitehead, M. (1988) *Inequalities in Health: The Black Report and the Health Divide*, Harmondsworth: Penguin.

Tuckett, D. (ed.) (1976) *An Introduction to Medical Sociology*, London: Tavistock.

Ungerson, C. (1987) *Policy is Personal*, London: Tavistock.

Vaus, D. A. de (1986) *Surveys in Social Research*, London: Allen & Unwin.

Victor, C. R. (1987) *Old Age in Modern Society, A Textbook of Social Gerontology*, London: Croom Helm.

Wagner, G. (Chairman) (1988) *Residential Care: A Positive Choice,* National

Institute for Social Work, London: HMSO.

Wald, N., Kiryluk, S., Darby, S., Doll, R., Pike, M. and Peto, R. (1988) *UK Smoking Statistics*, Oxford: Oxford University Press.

Walker, A. (1981) 'Towards a political economy of old age', *Ageing and Society*, 1 (1), 73–94.

Walker, A. (1983) 'Social policy and elderly people in Great Britain: the construction of dependent social and economic status in old age', in A. M. Guillemard (ed.) *Old Age and the Welfare State*, London: Sage.

Warnes, A. M. (1989) 'The ageing of populations', in A. Warnes (ed.) *Human Ageing and Later Life*, London: Edward Arnold.

Wells, N. E. J. (1979) *Dementia in Old Age*, London: Office of Health Economics.

Wells, N. and Freer, C. (eds) (1988) *The Ageing Population, Burden or Challenge?* London: Macmillan.

Wenger, G. C. (1984) *The Supportive Networks: coping with old age*, London: Allen & Unwin.

Wenger, G. C. (1986) 'What do dependency measures measure? Challenging assumptions', in C. Phillipson, H. Bernard and P. Strang (eds) *Dependency and Interdependence in Old Age*, London: Croom Helm, pp. 65–84.

Wenger, G. C. (1988) *Old People's Health and Experiences of the Caring Services*, Liverpool: The Institute of Human Ageing, Occ. Paper, Liverpool University Press.

West, P., Illsley, R. and Kelman, H. (1984) 'Public preferences for the care of dependency groups', *Social Science & Medicine*, 18 (4), 287–95.

Williams, R. (1986) 'Images of age & generation', Paper for *British Sociological Association Conference*, 1986.

Wilson, P. (1980) *Drinking in England and Wales*, London: HMSO.

Winter, J. M. (1985) *The Great War and the British People*, London: Macmillan.

WHO (1977) *Working Group on the Prevention of Mental Disorders in the Elderly*, Copenhagen: WHO.

Yorkshire Television (1987) 'The granny business', *First Tuesday* programme.

Young, M. (1988) *The Metronomic Society*, London: Thames & Hudson.

Young, M. and Willmott, P. (1957) *Family and Kinship in East London*, London: Routledge & Kegan Paul.

Zola, I. K. (1966) 'Culture and symptoms: an analysis of patients presenting complaints', *American Sociological Review*, 31, 615–30.

NAME INDEX

SUBJECT INDEX